Wellness 100

100 Carbs/100 Recipes

Amber French, DO

Kari Morris

http://wellness100.us

Published in the United States by BQB Publishing
(Boutique of Quality Books Publishing Company)
www.bqbpublishing.com

Printed in the United States of America

ISBN 978-1-937084-57-8 (p)
ISBN 978-1-937084-59-2 (h)
ISBN 978-1-937084-58-5 (e)

Library of Congress Control Number: 2012940555

Cover Illustration by Dan Edwards
Book design by Robin Krauss, www.lindendesign.biz
Photography by Jerry Morris

Acknowledgments

We would like to thank our husbands, Kevin French and Jerry Morris, for their support both in adopting the Wellness 100 lifestyle and of the huge time commitment required throughout the months of researching, writing, editing, cooking, and tasting the recipes that are represented in this book. To our families and friends, we are so appreciative of the continual encouragement you have shown and of your anticipation of the release of this book. It has been a long time coming, and you never failed to ask about our progress or share your enthusiasm for the data and the recipes. We hope *Wellness 100: 100 Carbs/100 Recipes* exceeds your expectations. We also want to thank the team at BQB Publishing. This young hybrid publishing company under the leadership of Terri Leidich is opening doors for new authors like us and changing the way quality books are brought to print in a digital age. Many thanks in particular to Terri, Julie, Katy, Jan, and Janet for their expertise, faith, patience, and professionalism.

Contents

A Word to You from Dr. Amber French

If you are reading this, you have decided to give up fad diets and do something really good for your body. The Wellness 100 program described in this book is designed to be a lifestyle change and a long-term solution—not just for weight loss, but for better overall health. The program is called Wellness 100 because we are sure that a diet of 100 carbohydrates per day will change your life. By following this program, you will be slowing down the changes that come with aging at the cellular level in your body. You will be preventing damage to your body that leads to heart disease, stroke, cancer, diabetes, and other diseases of aging. Getting to a healthier weight is just one of the beneficial effects of Wellness 100.

This program works exceptionally well for people with diabetes, high cholesterol, and existing heart disease. If you do not have one of those ailments, Wellness 100 will help prevent these types of problems. I have seen many cases where people can cut back or eliminate their medications altogether. I believe that the purpose of the medical profession is to prevent illness and aging. The core of wellness comes from good nutrition.

Wellness 100 is based on hundreds of research articles and books, not just a few of my observations or preferences. If I were designing a diet based on my unscientific personal preferences, it would be pasta for every meal, with bread and dessert, washed down with wine! I tried this, but it doesn't work!

In medical school, I was taught that "calories in and calories out" are the only things that matter for weight loss. But the reality is, it's not that simple, because a healthy lifestyle and a fit weight are more about the type of calories you consume than the amount of calories. For example, you may be able to lose weight in the short term with a low-calorie diet; but like most people, you will probably plateau at a certain point and not lose any more weight.

Imagine eating nothing but junk food, but staying under a thousand calories a day. You may initially lose weight, but you would be causing a lot of damage to your body by not getting the necessary food elements. In the short term, you would feel sluggish and have other vague health complaints due to the lack of vitamins, minerals, and beneficial calories in your food. The long-term effects would be worse, including diabetes, heart disease, cancers, and other diseases that not only shorten your life but also decrease the quality of life.

Healthy weight loss is one to two pounds per week. Wellness 100 is designed to be slow and steady. You may get faster results with a fad diet, but Wellness 100 will give you lasting results and a lifestyle you will want to continue.

I have been doing this program personally and with my patients for about three years with wonderful results. About a year ago, Kari Morris (the best chef I know) came to me and said that she wanted to create recipes to prove to people that healthy food can be varied and flavorful. So the first section of this book, by me, will explain how you can combine carbohydrates, fats, and proteins. This section will show you how to make good decisions in each of those three categories. It will explain how Wellness 100 improves overall health and longevity. The second part of this book, by Kari Morris, provides you with 100 recipes to get you started. At the end of the book in the appendices, you will find nutritional information about foods, plus a handy grocery checklist. You can also find more information at the website companion to this book, http://wellness100.us .

I am passionate about preventing illness. One obvious solution seems to be to use good nutrition to slow down aging and to help avoid diseases. By eating right, you feel good and look good. You may recall the cartoon in which carrots and celery are dancing and singing, "You are what you eat, from your head down to your feet." How true that is! But somehow many people neglect the very basics of nutrition. This program will take you back to those basics. I am excited that you have taken this important step for your health!

Wishing you wellness,
Dr. Amber French

You Can Do It!
The Wellness 100 Program

CHAPTER 1
Overview to Wellness 100

Wellness 100 is a lifestyle, not a quick diet. This program will teach you how to make good food choices to keep calories and carbohydrates balanced with healthy fat and protein. You should enjoy eating and not feel deprived while you follow this program. You will not find unreasonable meal plans or unsustainable restrictions. Likewise, you will not find shortcuts, pills, or shots that allow you to carry on with bad eating habits! Read on to discover how 100 carbohydrates per day will change your life. You will discover that thin and healthy are not the same thing.

Years ago, my mother called me with the news that one of her co-workers had suffered a heart attack. My mother was shocked that Susan (thin and apparently healthy) could have a heart condition. I, however, was not surprised. I have known Susan almost my entire life; and as a teenager, I remember marveling that Susan could eat fast-food and candy bars, drink soda all day, and never gain weight. As a physician, I know that those of us who put on weight when we eat like that are actually the lucky ones. Don't laugh! We get a warning sign that we are doing unhealthy things to our body. Our physical appearance can serve as a wake-up call to change our diet, so that we can prevent heart disease, diabetes, and other internal diseases of aging.

The first half of this book teaches you how to eat, and the second half contains recipes that are flavorful, satisfying, and meet the guidelines of Wellness 100. You will also find information at the website companion to this book, http://wellness100.us . I will explain each of the program's guidelines, which are shown in Table 1.1.

Calories Count: Both Minimum and Maximum

Counting calories is not just about losing weight. Wellness 100 is about living a long, healthy life. Fitting back into your skinny jeans may or may not happen. The minimum number of calories that healthy adults need to take in on a daily basis is 1,200 for women and 1,400 for men. Any fewer calories and the body behaves as if it is starving. A starving body reduces energy expenditure for basic bodily functions, and this metabolic adaptation reduces your rate of weight loss! Repeated cycles of severe caloric restriction or starvation cause an increase in food efficiency, which makes it harder to lose weight in the future. Essentially, your body gets confused and tries to hold on to all the energy (fat) that it can.

For example, Margaret had been dieting since she was a child. She confessed to me that when she was an adolescent and early teen, her father gave her weight-loss pills. She tried every diet imaginable and "yo-yoed" up and down with weight loss or gain for years. Now, at age 65, she is following this program. If she does not follow it exactly, she gains back everything she has lost. Her body has become overly efficient at storing her nutrients because of the years of cyclical starvation. Margaret provides an example of how years of bad dieting can make it harder to lose weight, even with this program, and why I do not recommend any fad diets, especially the extremely low-calorie ones.

Table 1.1
Wellness 100 Guidelines

100 grams of carbohydrates per day: 30 with each meal and 5 to 8 grams per snack	• Never eat carbohydrates alone; always include good fat and protein • Focus on low glycemic carbohydrates • No white food (potatoes, white rice, sugar, white flour, etc.)
Real foods only: no low-fat, no-fat, low-carbohydrate, pre-packaged, or processed foods	
A minimum of 70 grams of protein per day	• A serving of meat should be 4 to 6 ounces • Two (or more) servings of fish per week • A maximum of 10 grams of protein from dairy
Eat a salad a day; raw vegetables provide more nutrients than cooked vegetables	
Never eat trans fat, and limit saturated fats; use monounsaturated or polyunsaturated fats	• Include 2 tablespoons of olive oil per day in your diet
Drinks should include water and herbal teas (avoid sugary, caffeinated drinks and diet beverages)	
Caloric intake is based on height, age, and gender	• Divide calories between three balanced meals per day and, if needed, two balanced snacks
Exercise 2.5 hours per week; walking will suffice, but get up and out there for weight loss and maintenance	

If you want to be absolutely precise in your caloric needs to achieve weight loss, you can do a lot of complicated calculations. However, Table 1.2 gives you an accurate estimate. I arrived at these numbers by averaging basal metabolic rates within age/height range and with an average activity level, then factoring in a 15–20 percent caloric reduction.

Not surprisingly, some researchers now are exploring a possible set point for weight. You will notice that once you reach a certain weight, your body does not want to respond with weight loss, no matter what you do. This weight is most likely your body's set point. This set point is going to be a healthy weight, and the point will increase some as we age. Forget what you weighed in high school. Not only is that unrealistic, it is most likely an unhealthy goal. Losing too much weight also makes you look older as you lose the fat under the skin of your face. Is it attractive to have a 30-year-old body and a 100-year-old face? My point here is that we all need to find a comfortable set point for our weight. That is why you will not find a chart with ideal weights in this book. If you are happy with your weight—and more important, your blood sugar level—and your cholesterol numbers are good, that is a healthy weight for you.

Table 1.2
Daily Calories for Weight Loss Based on Gender, Age, and Height

Women	20 to 29	30 to 39	40 to 49	50 to 59	60+
4'10'	1,200	1,200	1,200	1,200	1,200
4'11'	1,210	1,210	1,210	1,210	1,210
5'0'	1,220	1,220	1,220	1,220	1,220
5'1'	1,230	1,230	1,230	1,230	1,230
5'2'	1,250	1,235	1,235	1,235	1,235
5'3'	1,275	1,240	1,240	1,240	1,240
5'4'	1,300	1,255	1,245	1,245	1,245
5'5'	1,330	1,280	1,250	1,250	1,250
5'6'	1,360	1,315	1,265	1,255	1,255
5'7'	1,290	1,340	1,290	1,260	1,260
5'8'	1,415	1,370	1,320	1,275	1,270
5'9'	1,445	1,400	1,350	1,300	1,280
5'10'	1,475	1,425	1,375	1,330	1,285
5'11'	1,500	1,450	1,405	1,350	1,300
6'0'	1,530	1,480	1,430	1,385	1,340

Men	20 to 29	30 to 39	40 to 49	50 to 59	60+
5'2'	1,445	1,400	1,400	1,400	1,400
5'3'	1,470	1,420	1,410	1,410	1,410
5'4'	1,500	1,455	1,420	1,420	1,420
5'5'	1,520	1,475	1,430	1,425	1,425
5'6'	1,550	1,500	1,450	1,430	1,430
5'7'	1,580	1,530	1,480	1,435	1,435
5'8'	1,600	1,560	1,510	1,460	1,445
5'9'	1,635	1,585	1,540	1,490	1,460
5'10'	1,660	1,615	1,565	1,520	1,470

Table continued

Men	20 to 29	30 to 39	40 to 49	50 to 59	60+
5'11'	1,700	1,640	1,600	1,545	1,500
6'0'	1,730	1,675	1,630	1,580	1,530
6'1'	1,760	1,710	1,660	1,615	1,565
6'2'	1,790	1,740	1,690	1,645	1,600
6'3'	1,820	1,775	1,725	1,680	1,630
6'4'	1,860	1,810	1,760	1,715	1,667

When to Stop Counting Calories

After you achieve your weight loss goal, you should be able to add back 20 percent more calories for weight maintenance. Most people following Wellness 100 will find that for weight maintenance, they do not have to count calories. If you continue to follow the recommendations regarding carbohydrate restrictions and guidelines for the program, the proteins and fats fall into place. If you reach a plateau during weight loss, you may be tempted to lower your calories but leave your carbohydrates the same. Do not do this. Instead, try varying the food in your diet or increasing your exercise. I advise this method with my patients, and it always works.

Caloric Restriction Is Tied to Longevity

Anti-aging research is proving that lowering the amount of calories you consume makes you live longer. The years gained are not characterized by poor health, but by a more youthful body. Eating fewer calories helps prevent cancer, heart disease, diabetes, autoimmune disorders, Alzheimer's, and many other diseases associated with aging.

Skeptical? Consider the Okinawans. They have one of the longest average lifespan in the world. On average, they eat 40 percent fewer calories than people in the United States and 17 percent fewer calories than mainland Japanese.

Carbohydrates

Carbohydrates are not off limits. In fact, you need carbs, but you need to consume them in moderation. To stay healthy, you need only 30 grams of carbohydrates per meal and 5 grams per snack, for a total of 100 grams per day. Your brain functions better on carbohydrates than it does on ketone bodies (breakdown products of fatty acids). You must feed your brain. When it comes to carbohydrates, this is not a contest to see "how low can you go." One hundred (100) carbohydrates per day is the right amount.

Always choose good carbohydrates. You should not plan a meal completely empty of carbohydrates, then wash it down with a cola. Add to your diet healthy carbohydrates with fiber, such as vegetables, fruit, or whole grains.

Fat

Most of us are terrified of the macronutrient known as fat. Forget what you have learned about fat. Chapter 3, on fat, will completely change the way you look at it in your diet. You do not need to count grams of fat, as long as they are from good sources. Healthy fats can be found in foods like lean meats, nuts, seeds, vegetable oils, and avocados. A perfect lunch is a salad topped with fresh vegetables, avocados, sunflower seeds, lean meat or fish, and olive oil. If you are a "low-fat dieter," this sounds like a lot of calories from fat. However, good fats are nothing to fear. We need to have them in our diet. Good fats actually lower our cholesterol. (That last line is a teaser to get you to read the chapter on fat!)

Protein

You will notice that the minimum requirement for protein (70 grams per day) is still less than the maximum requirement for carbohydrates (100 per day). Wellness 100 is designed to provide balance to your diet. The protein chapter in this book will explain why you need protein, and how it helps you lose weight if you choose the right sources of protein. Choose lean cuts of meat to avoid higher levels of saturated fat. Red meat is fine, but in moderation. Fish should be consumed twice per week at a minimum. Keep your daily consumption of dairy down to a moderate amount as well. (Please note, if you are a vegetarian, and you rely on cheese for large amounts of protein, you may need to add a protein powder to foods like smoothies or yogurt to increase your protein consumption.)

Seventy (70) grams of protein per day may sound like a high number if you are not used to eating it at every meal. But consider this example of a daily intake: two eggs have about 13 grams of protein, a 4-ounce chicken breast has 35 grams of protein, and 4 ounces of salmon has 25 grams of protein. The total is 73 grams of protein, without even counting it from other sources such as beans, nuts, and some vegetables. If you were to get all of your protein through meat only, you could do so by eating only 8 to 9 ounces per day.

Meals

In a perfect world, we would all follow the adage, "Breakfast like a king, lunch like a prince, and dinner like a pauper." But we don't live in a perfect world. In the morning, we are in a hurry to get to work or school, or get others to work or school. We don't take the time to have a leisurely lunch. Dinner is usually our only opportunity to sit down and enjoy a meal. I have designed this program with a practical approach in mind.

Breakfast

You must eat breakfast. I repeat, you must eat breakfast, and coffee with cream does not count. You should be hungry in the morning; if you are not, it may be because you have trained your body not to be. Breakfast sets the tone for your body's metabolism for the rest of the day.

You need to consume 20 to 30 percent of your total calories for the day in the morning. These calories can come from breakfast and, if necessary, a midmorning snack. Do not feel obligated to snack if you are not hungry. From the calorie chart in Table 1.2, you can see that the minimum amount of calories for breakfast for anyone following this program is 250 (20 percent of 1,200). Only 120 of those calories can be from carbohydrates (30 carbs x 4 calories per carb = 120). So at the minimum, half of your breakfast calories must come from protein and fat.

Breakfast is the hardest meal to break out of the carbohydrate rut. Remember to think outside the box (the cereal box); and, as you will learn later in this book, embrace the egg! Lean cuts of meat are also a good choice for breakfast. This program is not a bacon-and-eggs-for-breakfast type of program. Bacon is not a lean meat, and it should be eaten in moderation. There are other protein options for breakfast, and Chapter 10 is dedicated to recipes to help you make the right choices for your first meal of the day.

Lunch

Lunch (and, if necessary, an afternoon snack) should contain 30 to 40 percent of your calories for the day. Plan and think ahead for lunch to avoid the pitfall of reaching for convenience foods like fast food or frozen meals loaded with sodium, preservatives, and extra carbohydrates. When making dinner at night, cook a little extra to take for lunch the next day. On weekends, make a soup and eat it for lunch on Monday and Tuesday. Keep a variety of salad ingredients on hand so that you can always take a salad. Keep olive oil at work so that you have a good dressing option, even if you have to run out to buy a salad. Try going to a grocery store salad bar for lunch, instead of a fast-food drive-through. You can always buy veggies off the salad bar and a container of hummus, with maybe a little bit of lunch meat for protein.

Dinner

The remaining 30 to 40 percent of your calories should be consumed with dinner. Meat, vegetable, and starch for dinner—that's how I was raised, and I'm sure a lot of you were, too. If you are like me, the starch was your favorite, and often the biggest portion on your plate. I find the easiest way to stay within the program guidelines at dinner is to plan your main protein, plan your vegetables, and then plan other healthy carbohydrates to add up to 30 grams. If the rest of your family doesn't want to eat the way that you are eating, that is okay. You can usually cook whatever you would normally cook for dinner and just modify it a little. If you make tacos, make yours into a taco salad. Whole wheat pasta can be a side dish, not a main course. And remember, fruit makes a wonderful sweet treat after dinner.

Finally, try to eat dinner early. Studies show that fasting for twelve hours overnight promotes weight loss.

Snacks

If you are hungry between meals, please have a snack. Snacks should be limited to 100 calories and 5 to 8 grams of carbohydrates. The temptation will be to grab a piece of fruit—fruit is good for you, right? Right, but not by itself. Fruits are carbohydrates. For the most part, they are good carbohydrates, packed with fiber and vitamins; but fruits are still carbohydrates. You can have fruit but make sure it is always paired with good fat and protein and limited to 5 to 8 grams of carbs. In this book, you will find a lot of helpful information on snacks.

Drinks

Drinks are a hidden danger. In the South, people often have sweet tea at every meal. This sugar-caffeine drink is difficult for my patients to give up. One 12-ounce glass of sweet tea may contain 27 grams of carbs (108 calories) or more from sugar. A regular can of soda has about 40 grams of carbs. Cocktails are even worse; a margarita can have as many calories as a Big Mac.

Eat most of your calories rather than drinking them, and you will be more satisfied. Drink more water, and replace many of your bad beverages during the day with herbal tea. If you want something flavored, try cutting fruit juice 50/50 with sparkling water; but only do this with a meal.

I don't recommend diet beverages for two reasons. First, the caffeine in most of them causes a temporary increase in the serotonin in your brain. You feel good, but then you crash. When the crash comes, you reach for either more caffeine or sugar to give you another boost. This is why people don't lose weight drinking diet beverages. Second, most artificial sweeteners are fairly toxic to our bodies (more on that in Chapter 6, "Hidden Calories and Hidden Dangers"). If you crave a soda, I would rather you drink a small amount of the real thing rather than the diet variety.

Wine with dinner is fine if you count the carbohydrates. A 4-ounce glass of red wine has about 100 calories, and the equivalent of 8 carbohydrates. Alcohol sugars are calculated a different way. Red wine, however, is the only alcohol with any health benefits. If you are going to drink anything else, remember to do so in moderation, and realize that it will affect your carbohydrate count and calories.

Drinking milk is not as necessary for calcium consumption as you may think. You can get enough calcium in your diet from other sources, such as broccoli and other green, leafy vegetables. You will learn later in this book why you don't really need to drink milk.

Salads

Did you know that french fries make up 25 percent of all vegetables consumed by Americans? As a society, we obviously are not making good vegetable choices. Eating one salad per day is a great way to get more vegetables, particularly raw vegetables, into your diet. Salads are also a great delivery method for the olive oil that I want you to consume (see the information that follows). Salads can either be an entrée or a side dish. Be creative! Chapter 11 is dedicated entirely to salad recipes.

Olive Oil

Olive oil is good for your heart. Studies on the Mediterranean diet have found that 2 tablespoons of olive oil per day is cardio-protective. It is a rich source of good fat in the form of monounsaturated fatty acids. (More on MUFAs in Chapter 3.) Olive oil also contains antioxidants, which have been shown to lower blood pressure and cholesterol. It is rich in vitamins E and K, and substances in olive oil may also be protective against Alzheimer's disease. It is perfect to cook with, because it is heat stable, which means that the fats found in olive oil do not change into bad or unhealthy fats when heated for cooking.

One last fun fact about olive oil: Like wine, the taste of olive oil is influenced not only by the olive, but also by where it is grown. Olive oil from Italy doesn't taste the same as olive oil from Spain, even if the same olives are used. Taste has to do with the soil type and the climate, known in wine-making as "terroir."

Exercise

How much exercise do you need in order to lose weight and maintain weight? That question is not easily answered. After researching this topic thoroughly for my patients, I can say that the magic number seems to be 2.5 hours per week for weight loss and some amount of time less than that for maintenance. Your exercise does not need to be hours of running. Any motion that gets your heart rate up will work as exercise. Walking is perfect, and it not as hard on your knees as running. Exercise is heart healthy, too. It will raise your HDL (good cholesterol) and lower your blood pressure.

I recommend to those patients who don't already exercise, to do so an hour each day of the weekend, or whatever their days off may be; then they should find one other day to squeeze-in some exercise. Doing it this way is not as optimal as spreading it out through the week, but it is a better plan than no plan. If you find yourself saying that you just can't find the time, ask yourself how many hours each day you watch television. That usually puts exercise time into perspective.

By now you should have a firm grasp of what you should do. The remainder of this book should enlighten you as to why the guidelines work, and it will provide you with the tools to make this lifestyle change easier than you think it may be.

CHAPTER 2
100 Carbohydrates a Day

Diet advice has run to the extremes for years. We have forgotten the wisdom of happy mediums. Clear your mind from things you may have heard about dieting, such as "all fat is bad," "carbohydrates are evil," and "whatever you do, stay away from red meat!" What has this so-called "wisdom" accomplished? It has left us with chemically altered food containing little to no nutritional value and certainly no flavor. Balance is the key, and after years of research and treating patients, I find the most effective way to achieve balance is to count the carbohydrates and let the protein and fat fall into place. It is easy to remember 100 grams of carbohydrates per day. It is harder to overdo it on protein and fat, because they are more filling than carbohydrates.

Points to Remember about Carbohydrates

- *Aim for 30 grams of carbs with each meal.*
- *No more than 5 to 8 grams of carbs in a 100-calorie snack.*
- *Never eat carbs alone.* Always eat carbs with good fat and protein.
- *Fruits are mostly carbs.*
- *Save enough carbs for some fruit in your diet.*
- *Avoid fruit juices.* They have a higher glycemic index than the fruit, and the fiber is gone.
- *Try to consume only the good carbs (no white food).*
- *Choose foods with a lower glycemic index.*
- *Eat whole grains.*
- *Choose brown or wild rice, not white rice.*
- *Keep sugar to a bare minimum;* and if you need a sweetener use honey, agave, stevia, or truvia.
- *Desserts are not an everyday treat.*
- *Never use artificial sweeteners containing aspartame.*

Guidelines for Eating Carbohydrates

Always eat carbohydrates with good fat and protein. Never eat carbohydrates alone. Eating carbohydrates alone will make you fat! I cannot stress enough how important this fact is to your overall health. Each meal should include 30 grams of carbohydrates, and each snack should have 5 to 8 grams of carbohydrates, giving you about 100 grams of carbohydrates per day.

Weight Loss

Most head-to-head studies of low-carbohydrate and low-fat diets show that they are about equal on weight-loss results. Either diet with a calorie restriction will help you to lose weight. For health reasons, however, a low-carbohydrate diet is preferable to a low-fat diet.

- The evidence supports the lessening of a cardiovascular risk and a diabetes risk with a Mediterranean-style, low-carbohydrate diet such as this program.
- Weight loss with a low-carbohydrate diet is concentrated around the middle section. As long as you keep your protein content high enough, you will retain lean muscle mass while you lose weight.
- You will keep the weight off—if, once you go back up on your calories, you keep the protein content high and maintain 100 carbs a day.

100 Grams of Carbohydrates

How did I choose the magic number of 30 grams of carbohydrates with each meal? Why not calculate a percentage? How can it be the same for everyone? The answer is that no diet is perfect for everyone, but most studies involving low carbohydrates and their benefits keep this number at 100 grams or below.

Hundreds of studies examine the effects of carbohydrates on blood sugar, cholesterol, triglycerides, and weight loss. The most effective of the diets that were studied used amounts of carbohydrates at or below 100 grams per day, or 30 percent of the diet. Given that no one following Wellness 100 should eat less than 1,200 calories per day, and each gram of carbohydrate has 4 calories, we can do the math. So, 30 + 30 + 30 + 10 for snacks = 100 grams of carbohydrates × 4 calories = 400, which is 33 percent of a 1,200 calorie diet.

Let's say that your caloric recommendation is more than 1,200 calories per day. Does that mean you get more carbs? Sorry, but no. Again, this program is not based on personal opinion or preference; it is based on scientific evidence that shows that a low-carbohydrate diet is 100 grams of carbohydrates per day in order to have the observed health benefits.

Counting grams of carbs rather than figuring a percentage based on your caloric intake is much easier to learn and stick with. Once you know your carbs and have a basic understanding of the compositions of the foods you eat, this method becomes second nature.

This program probably is not perfect for everyone. (Bet you didn't see that line coming!) So many diet books claim, "This is it, this is the way everyone should eat." I am more open minded than that. There are a lot of ways to lose weight. Wellness 100 is more than a diet; it is a lifestyle. Of course, one goal is to help you lose weight; but in the bigger picture, Wellness 100 will help you stay thin and live a healthier, longer life. Variations from person to person, both genetic and environmental, influence the way that individuals metabolize carbohydrates, fats, and proteins. Thus it's not possible to design a program that is perfect for everyone. What I promise is that Wellness 100 works for almost everyone and will not cause diabetes and heart disease while you lose weight, as some other weight-loss programs might.

What Is a Carbohydrate?

Essentially, anything sugary or starchy is a carbohydrate. Any food with a sugary or starchy component has carbohydrates in it. A carbohydrate is one of three macronutrients, as are fat and protein. The term carbohydrate is synonymous with saccharide. There are four general groupings: monosaccharides, disaccharides, oligosaccharides, and polysaccharides. Monosaccharides and disaccharides are usually referred to as "sugar." Sugar is simply a carbohydrate in its simplest form.

Carbohydrates Make You Hungry

I skipped breakfast for twenty years, because eating breakfast always made me hungry. Does this sound familiar? The idea of a healthy breakfast with cereal and milk, a piece of fruit, and a glass of fruit juice is a sugar bomb. This type of meal would give you a rush of sugar; and when the spike of blood sugar comes down, it leaves you hungry for more. Sugar temporarily increases the serotonin in your brain, which makes you feel happy. Then, when the serotonin drops again, you reach for something to make you feel good. Your brain craves another rush of sugar or caffeine, which can do the same thing. Coffee and doughnuts, anyone?

Breakfast seems to be the hardest meal to beat the carbohydrate rut. Think outside the box (the cereal box!) of what is typically considered breakfast food, or at least what people in the United States consider breakfast food. In other parts of the world, meats and cheeses are usually consumed for breakfast. Don't be afraid to wrap your leftovers from the night before in a corn tortilla and walk out the door in the morning. Learn to love eggs again (not egg substitutes, and not just the egg whites).

Egg substitutes contain about 99 percent egg whites and 1 percent natural flavoring. Nutrients are added back into the egg substitutes to make up for those taken out with the yolks. Real eggs have about 5 grams of fat and only 2 to 3 grams of saturated fat. As you will read in Chapter 3, thirty years of research on the cholesterol in eggs has failed to show an association between eggs and heart disease. The type of cholesterol found in eggs actually makes your body's cholesterol better for you. You can use egg substitutes if you want, but when the real thing is so good for you, why bother?

Replacing Carbohydrates with Good Fat and Protein

Obviously, if you decrease your carbohydrate intake, then you will need to make up the calories somewhere else. Be careful with your replacement calories. Just as with carbohydrates, not all fat and protein are equally good for you. Unfortunately, the low-fat craze did not distinguish between trans fat, saturated fats, monounsaturated fatty acids (MUFA), and polyunsaturated fatty acids (PUFA). We will address the differences between these fats in Chapter 3, which is dedicated to them; but suffice it to say that as long as you replace the carbohydrate calories with MUFA and PUFA (not trans fats and saturated fats), you do not increase your risk for heart disease. Similarly, you must be careful about your choice of protein. You want to pick meat sources of protein that are lean and to eat a strictly controlled amount of dairy. You are not following this program if you go to a fast-food restaurant, order a triple bacon cheeseburger, and then eat it without the bun!

Choosing the Right Carbohydrates

Another danger is choosing empty carbohydrates instead of carbohydrates with the vitamins and minerals that you need. French fries are not good carbohydrates. The temptation is to get very excited about the 30 grams of carbohydrates you can have with each meal and not plan for the right ones. For example, perhaps you decide that your carbohydrates are going to be the not-so-good-for-you potato or pasta and then forget to eat fruit. Save room for the good carbohydrates, such as fruits and whole grains. I see this problem with my patients all the time. Please do not think that fruits are bad and that you shouldn't eat them. Fruits are wonderful and should be part of your diet, but you cannot have a potato for dinner and then eat a bowl of fruit for dessert. You will have to choose one or the other.

Once my patients get started on Wellness 100, many comment that they find it hard to get carbohydrates in their diet. Once again, do not forget the fruit. Fruits are the perfect answer and are for the most part "good" carbohydrates. If you realize that your breakfast didn't have 30 grams of carbohydrates, add a piece of fruit. If you want a sweet treat after dinner, add fruit. Fruits have fiber and lots of vitamins. Keep a variety of fruits on hand to complement any meal.

Apples are easy to keep around because they typically don't go bad fast. Do not store apples with any other fruits or vegetables unless you are trying to ripen those foods quickly. Apples contain an enzyme that will ripen any other fruit that they are stored next to.

The easiest way to plan a meal is to plan your main dish, plan a vegetable or two (including a salad), and then count the carbohydrates. You then can add in more carbohydrates to make up the difference to 30 grams. Experience with my patients has taught me to repeat this advice as many times as I can. If you get very excited about eating something with carbohydrates in your meal, like pasta, and then try to plan the rest of your meal around this carbohydrate "core," you will go over! The end of this chapter has some information on the carbohydrates that you can add to your meal.

What Good Things Do Carbohydrates Do?

This diet is not an anti-carbohydrate program. Carbohydrates are necessary and vital to many of your body's functions. Your brain and nervous system function much better on carbohydrates than they do on ketone bodies (breakdown products of fatty acids used for energy in the absence of carbohydrates). If you do not give your brain enough "sugar," you will feel foggy. A diet totally empty of carbohydrates can cause fatigue, insomnia, depression, and headaches. Your brain has no storage capacity for glucose, so the body must have a constant supply. You cannot cut them out of your diet completely, but you can cut them down to a safer, healthier amount.

Fiber is a carbohydrate that cannot be digested. Fiber is good for your cholesterol and decreases the glycemic index (sugar rush) of each meal. It is also important for colon health. Without carbohydrates, you will get very little fiber in your diet. If you find that you are not getting enough fiber, you can always drink a psyllium-based fiber drink (without sugar) in the morning. It will also make you feel fuller, and thus help you to eat less.

Carbohydrates and Disease

With the advent of improved sanitation, safer working environments, modern surgery, and safer childbearing, more people are now living long enough to deal with age-related health issues such as heart disease and diabetes. So how do carbohydrates contribute to the biggest killers we face?

HDL is our good cholesterol, right? (There is more information on cholesterol in Chapter 3.) A carbohydrate-rich diet lowers our good cholesterol. Low-fat foods that you may think are healthy actually make it worse. Most fat-free foods replace the naturally occurring fat with carbohydrates to make it taste better. Ask yourself—Is it really necessary to have a dozen fat-free cookies a day, anyway? (I'm talking about those hundred-calorie snack packs.) Wouldn't it make more sense just to save the cookie or dessert for special occasions, instead of making it part of your daily diet?

The evidence is overwhelming that a high-carbohydrate diet lowers our HDL, the "good cholesterol," and raises our LDL, or "bad" cholesterol. If that evidence isn't bad enough, we have learned that not all "bad" cholesterol is created equal. The type of cholesterol that is made when you eat a high-carbohydrate diet is worse for you.

Studies also show that a high-carbohydrate diet increases triglycerides. For women, high triglycerides more accurately predict heart disease than does one's total cholesterol. One of the best ways to lower triglycerides is to have a diet high in MUFA (monounsaturated fatty acids). I know this advice goes against everything that you may have heard about your cholesterol levels. My patients and even the occasional colleague are constantly amazed that following Wellness 100 (eating eggs and meat, while cutting out the sugar) improves their cholesterol numbers.

Carbohydrates Affect Blood Sugar and Insulin

When you eat fewer carbohydrates, your blood sugar levels go down. This strategy will decrease your risk for developing diabetes and the associated plaqueing of the arteries leading to heart disease. If you suffer from hypoglycemia and feel that you need sugar to avoid getting dizzy, eating a low, balanced, carbohydrate diet will keep blood sugars more stable. Without the peaks and valleys of fluctuating blood sugar, you will feel better.

A low-carbohydrate diet improves insulin sensitivity. If you are diabetic, limiting

Insulin is a hormone secreted by your pancreas that causes the cells in your liver, muscles, and fat tissue to take up glucose (sugar) from your blood. Type 1 diabetics do not make enough insulin. Type 2 diabetics are not able to use their insulin effectively, because the cells in their bodies have become resistant to insulin. Their bodies then make more insulin to try to compensate.

your carbs will put less sugar into your system. The sugar/carbohydrates that do make it into your system will be taken up into your cells faster, using less insulin. You can lower your insulin requirement by adhering to a low-carbohydrate diet.

Insulin is the biggest hormone that triggers your liver to make cholesterol. High insulin levels in response to a high-carbohydrate diet and high–glycemic-index meals induce the liver to overproduce cholesterol. More carbohydrates in your diet equals more insulin, which equals more cholesterol. And, as stated previously, this type of cholesterol is worse for you.

Simple vs. Complex Carbohydrates, or Good vs. Evil (It Is Not that Simple)

Not all simple carbohydrates are bad, and not all complex carbohydrates are good. Simple carbohydrates include both table sugar and fruit. Obviously, the fruit has health benefits in the form of fiber and vitamins. In comparison, table sugar does not have such benefits. Simple carbohydrates are broken down faster in the body and provide a more immediate source of energy. Complex carbohydrates can be thought of as starches, and these can be found in white bread and vegetables. They are broken down more slowly and typically have a lower glycemic index (GI). Notice that I said typically, because white bread has a very high GI. So which do you think you should eat: the apple or the white bread? I hope you answered the apple. You should consume both simple and complex carbohydrates, but make sure that you are making good choices within those categories. To help you make those good choices, you need to understand a little bit about the glycemic index.

Glycemic Index

The glycemic index (GI) ranks foods on how quickly they raise our blood sugar. The concept was developed by Dr. David J. Jenkins and his colleagues in 1980–1981 at the University of Toronto. They were researching which foods are best for people with diabetes. The GI of a food is based on the blood sugar response to that food. The response to the test food is then given a number, based on how it ranks on a graph. This number gives a relative ranking for each tested food. The standard by which all others are measured is pure glucose, which at 100 has the highest glycemic index. Table sugar is composed of one molecule of glucose and one molecule of fructose, giving it a glycemic index of 75.

The glycemic index divides foods with carbohydrates into high, medium, and low values. A high glycemic index is 70 or greater. Medium GI is 55–69, and low is 54 or below. Please see the tables in this chapter for examples.

So why is this number important? The GI should guide your choice of which carbohydrates to include in your diet. When you eat something with a higher GI, like a donut, your blood sugar rises faster, increasing the insulin released by your body.

Higher levels of blood sugar lead to advanced glycation endproducts (AGEs), which cause physical signs of aging such as wrinkles, stiff joints, and glaucoma. Higher levels of insulin again stimulate the liver to produce cholesterol. Insulin is also damaging to the lining of our blood vessels, causing plaqueing of the arteries and heart disease.

Many things affect the glycemic index of a food. For example, higher fiber content will lower the glycemic index of an entire meal. Fiber increases the transit time through the gut, effectively making your meal "time-released" and lowering the amount of sugar that gets into your system at one time. This increased transit time provides a steadier state of blood sugar levels and a lower spike of insulin release. This fact is one of the dangers of juicing. When most people juice, they are throwing away the fiber and essentially just drinking a big infusion of sugar.

So, back to the apple: Is it better to have the whole apple, or the apple juice? Of course, the apple is better. I don't recommend fruit juice in general. You are much better off just eating a piece of fruit. After you have been on the program, even the no-sugar-added juices will seem too sweet to you. If you are really thirsty for a glass of juice, mix it fifty-fifty with some sparkling water. Don't forget to consume some good fat and protein with it.

Texture also influences the glycemic index. For example, coarse-ground flour has a lower GI than finely milled flour. The same is true for oatmeal. Steel-cut oats are less refined, and so this food spends a longer time in your gut being broken down. This longer transit time in the gut lowers the GI. Cooking methods also affect the glycemic index. For instance, baking seems to raise the GI of potatoes, whereas boiling lowers it.

Atherosclerosis is a condition in which an artery wall becomes thickened, narrowing the artery. The terms plaqueing, funneling, narrowing, and hardening of the arteries all mean the same thing. Cardiovascular disease (CVD) is caused by atherosclerosis. Coronary heart disease is when the narrowing occurs in the vessels supplying oxygen-rich blood to the heart.

The GI of pasta depends a lot upon the shape of the pasta; thicker pasta has lower GI. Like the GI of potatoes, the GI of pasta is influenced by how long it is cooked. When a person cooks pasta as the Italians cook it, al dente—somewhat firm—then it has a lower glycemic index. The longer you cook pasta, the mushier it gets, and the higher the GI. Notice I said "mushier" rather than "softer," because the Italians will tell you overcooked pasta is a culinary crime.

In addition to fiber, vinegar and alcohol can lower the GI of a meal. Drinking an alcoholic beverage before a meal may decrease the GI of the entire meal by up to 15 percent. Please do not use this fact as an excuse to drink more. If you do, you will consume too many calories and carbohydrates.

Be careful not to confuse grams of carbohydrates with the glycemic index. Just because a serving of white rice and a serving of brown rice have the same amount of carbohydrates, doesn't mean that they are equally good for you. The 30 grams of carbohydrates from the white rice are going to raise your blood sugar much more quickly, and higher, than the 30 grams of carbohydrates from the brown rice. Health benefits are not equal just because calorie and carbohydrate counts are equal.

Use Table 2.1 to identify low, medium, and high GI value foods. Include more low and medium GI foods in your diet.

Table 2.1
GI Values for Common Carbohydrate Food Sources*
Rated Low (< 55), Medium (56 to 69), and High (70+)

Fruits					
Low		**Medium**		**High**	
Cherries, sour	22	Papaya	56	Watermelon	72
Grapefruit	25	Raisins	56	Dates, dried	103
Prunes	29	Apricots, fresh	57		
Apricots, dried	30	Kiwi	58		
Apple	38	Figs, dried	61		
Pear	38	Cantaloupe	65		
Plum	39	Pineapple, fresh	66		
Strawberries	40				
Orange, navel	42				
Peach	42				
Grapes	46				
Mango	51				
Banana	52				

Vegetables					
Low		**Medium**		**High**	
Most vegetables (asparagus, artichokes, bell pepper, broccoli, Brussels sprouts, cabbage, cauliflower, celery, cucumbers, eggplant, green beans, lettuce, mushrooms, onions, summer squash, tomatoes, zucchini)	22	Beets	64	Most potatoes	72
Carrots	47	Sweet potato	61	Mashed potatoes	74
Green peas	48			Pumpkin	75
Yam	51			French fries	75
Sweet corn	54			Russet potato, baked	85
				Instant mashed potato	85
				Parsnip	97

Breads and Crackers					
Low		Medium		High	
Pumpernickel	50	Pita, whole wheat	57	White bread	70
Corn tortilla	52	Rye crispbread	64	Most crackers	103
Sourdough	53	Taco shell	68	Water crackers	71
Stone-ground, whole wheat	53			White bagel	72
				Baguette	95

Legumes (Beans)					
Low		Medium		High	
Chickpeas, dried	28				
Kidney beans, dried	28				
Lentils, green, dried	29				
Black beans	30				
Lima beans (frozen)	32				
Chickpeas, canned	42				
Black-eyed peas, canned	42				
Baked beans	48				
Kidney beans, canned	52				

Pasta					
Low		Medium		High	
Fettuccini (egg)	32	Rice vermicelli	58		
Spaghetti, whole wheat	37	Couscous	65		
Spaghetti, white (boiled 5 minutes)	38				
Spaghetti, white (boiled 10–15 minutes)	44				
Spiral pasta	43				
Linguine	46				
Macaroni	47				

Rice and Other Grains					
Low		Medium		High	
Barley, pearled	25	Quinoa	53	White rice, instant	87
		Brown rice	55		

Table continued

Rice and Other Grains					
Low		**Medium**		**High**	
		Wild rice	57		
		White rice, average	64		
		Cornmeal	68		

Dairy					
Low		**Medium**		**High**	
Whole milk	31	Ice cream, regular	61		
Skim milk	32				
Yogurt, sweetened	33				
Ice cream, premium	38				

Juice					
Low		**Medium**		**High**	
Tomato	38	Cranberry juice cocktail	68		
Apple	40				
Pineapple	46				
Grapefruit	48				
Orange	53				

Snacks					
Low		**Medium**		**High**	
Hummus	6	Power bar (chocolate)	56	Popcorn, microwave	72
Peanuts	14	Potato chips	57	Rice cakes	78
Walnuts	15	Corn chips	63	Pretzels	83
Cashews	22				
M&M peanut candies	33				
Milk chocolate	43				

*Source: International Table of Glycemic Index and Glycemic Load Values: 2002, American Journal of Clinical Nutrition, The American Society of Clinical Nutrition and The University of Sydney (www.glycemicindex.com)

Avoid the White Foods

Potatoes, white rice, white bread, and so forth all have higher glycemic indexes. Remember that simple carbohydrates and a high glycemic index are not synonymous.

Fructose found in fruits is a simple carbohydrate, but some fruits have a low glycemic index. Whole grains, brown rice, and lower glycemic fruits and vegetables are always going to be a healthier choice. When in doubt about whether a carbohydrate is good for you or not, think about the way nature intended the carbohydrate you want to eat. Does grain straight out of the field make white bread? No. Fruit, however, is in its natural state. What about potatoes? Okay, you got me on potatoes; you just have to make an exception. Even in their natural state, they are a higher GI food. That fact doesn't mean you can't ever eat them. Just eat them in moderation and make sure you keep the number under 30 grams of carbohydrates with each meal. That strategy doesn't leave a lot of room for potatoes.

Side Effects of a High-Carbohydrate Diet

As I began the process of editing this chapter, a patient (Linda) came into my office who put into perspective why I am offering you this book, and why I routinely discuss nutrition with my patients. Linda came in for a routine annual exam. I noticed in her chart that last year she complained of fatigue. Before I could ask for an update, she cut me off and said, "Dr. French, I didn't believe you when you told me that what I was eating was making me tired. When you told me last year to cut down on my carbohydrates and add more protein, I had no intention of doing that. But as the weeks went by, I felt so bad that I thought I may as well try it. I have to apologize for not believing you, because you were right. I feel so much better." Incidentally, she also lost 10 pounds. So remember that every facet of your health is influenced by your diet.

Carbohydrates affect your body in ways that you can't see or feel, but also carbs affect you in several ways that you can feel. For example, too many carbohydrates can cause heartburn. They can cause increased salt retention in the kidneys, which can cause swelling and lead to elevated blood pressure. A single meal that is heavy in carbohydrates can be too much for the stomach to handle, and some carbs will get to the small intestine undigested, where they will ferment, causing gas. And don't forget about those side effects caused by AGEs; they cause wrinkles and other signs and symptoms of aging.

Carbohydrates and Insulin

When you eat carbohydrates by themselves, insulin is released from your pancreas. Insulin's job is to make sure that sugar and amino acids get into the cells of your body. When you add protein to carbohydrates, not only do you decrease the glycemic index of the meal, but you also induce the pancreas to release glucagon.

Glucagon is a hormone that is often described as having the opposite action as insulin. Both are released from the pancreas at a basal or steady level, but the minute-to-minute variation in the amount of insulin or glucagon released is dependent on the carbohydrate and protein content of our meals. Insulin causes glucose to be stored as either energy or, if there is too much "sugar," as fat. So in general, insulin promotes the storage of glucose.

Glucagon is released by the pancreas and has metabolic actions on the liver, kidney, intestinal smooth muscle, brain, and adipose tissue. One action of glucagon is to mobilize sugar into the blood stream in response to hypoglycemia (low blood sugar). A meal with the right balance of carbohydrates and protein will cause more glucagon to be released from the pancreas. This method will not only help maintain a steady level of blood sugar, it will also help mobilize glucose from your liver and adipose tissue (fat).

It is an oversimplification to say that insulin is bad and glucagon is good. We need both, but when you adjust your diet to enhance the release of glucagon, this adjustment will help your body release stored energy from fat cells, helping you to lose weight.

Caution about Plateaus

As you lose weight, you will, at times, hit a plateau. What I have seen my patients do when this happens is that they decrease their calories, but they leave their carbohydrate consumption the same. Because this program is about balance, this method doesn't work. Don't do it. Just stay the course, and try varying your diet a little or intensifying your exercise routine.

Take-Home Message from this Chapter

Not all carbohydrates are evil. Wellness 100 is a balanced carbohydrate program, not a plan that is anti-carbohydrate or no-carbohydrate. Never eat carbohydrates alone; instead, eat 30 grams of carbohydrates per meal, always balanced with good fat and protein. Table 2.2 shows you the add-in carbs for meals. Use the glycemic index to help guide your carbohydrate choices. You are on this diet not just to lose weight, but also to improve your overall health. What do I mean by "good fat and protein"? Read on!

Table 2.2

Add-in Carbs for Meals

Carbohydrate Options	Amount	Grams of Carbs	Calories
Whole wheat pita	6 ½-inch diameter	35.2 grams	170
Couscous (cooked)	½ cup	18 grams	78.5
Brown rice (cooked)	½ cup	22.9 grams	109
Wild rice (cooked)	½ cup	17.5 grams	83
Whole grain bread	1 slice	20 grams	100
Ezekiel bread	1 slice	15 grams	80
Whole wheat English muffin	1 muffin	25 grams	130
Apple	1 medium	25.1 grams	95
Pear	1 medium	25.7 grams	96
Blueberries	1 cup	21.5 grams	84
Sweet potato (baked)	1 small 2.1 ounce	12.4 grams	54
White potato (baked)	1 small 4.9 ounce	29.3 grams	128
Flour tortilla	1 small	13 grams	90
Corn tortilla	1 small	10.7 grams	52
Whole wheat spaghetti	3 ounces (cooked)	22.5 grams	105
Risotto	¼ cup	31.5 grams	142.5
Quinoa (cooked with water)	½ cup	23.5 grams	127
Red wine	5 ounce	5.5 grams/12.5 grams of alcohol	127
Black beans	½ cup	20.4 grams	114

CHAPTER 3
We Need Fat

Fats are a source of energy to the body. It is unfortunate that we equate the fat in our diet with the fat around our middle, thighs, buttocks, and so on. Fat has been vilified because of the three macronutrients, it is the densest in calories. For example, carbohydrates and protein provide only 4 calories per gram, whereas fat has 9 calories per gram.

Fats are composed of mixture fatty acids. Fatty acids can be broadly divided into three categories based on their chemical structure, and, thus, their effect on the body. The three categories are unsaturated fatty acids, which include both monounsaturated (MUFA) and polyunsaturated (PUFA); saturated fatty acids; and trans fatty acids. This chapter will calm your fears about fat and cholesterol, and it will explain the scientific reasons why not all fats and cholesterol are harmful. Many of these are actually healthy and necessary.

The Truth about Fats and Cholesterol

- *Unsaturated fatty acids (MUFAs and PUFAs) are cardioprotective*
  These are found in nuts, olive oil, avocados, and some meats.

- *Saturated fats may not be all bad*
  Substitute with MUFA and PUFA when you can (for example, olive oil for butter).

  Eat leaner cuts of meat to cut back on saturated fat.

- *Trans fats are the enemy*
  There is no acceptable level of trans fats.

  They are human-made fats, so your body doesn't know what to do with them.

  These are foods that logically should not have a long shelf life, but suspiciously do.

  For example, you will see that some foods, like cookies from a vending machine, do have a long shelf life. This is a clue to you that you shouldn't eat it.
  Trans fats are found most commonly in snack foods and fast food.

  They raise our bad cholesterol.

- *Cholesterol in food doesn't change your blood cholesterol as much as you think*
  Cholesterol in the food we eat does very little to our blood cholesterol levels.

Wellness 100 does not count grams of fat. When you get the correct amount of carbohydrates in your diet and choose the right types of protein and fat, it all falls into place. For weight-loss purposes, you will be counting the calories that you get from fat. But you will find that it is much harder to go over on your calories for the day when you are feeling more satisfied and energetic from the proper amount of dietary fat and protein.

A common misconception is that dietary fat raises cholesterol. The biggest switch to turn on cholesterol production in the liver is insulin. And what makes insulin rise in our bloodstream? Carbohydrates! We will discuss cholesterol later in this chapter; but suffice it to say, not all fats raise cholesterol, and not all cholesterol in our diet is bad.

Omega 9, 6, 3 Fatty Acids

What are Omega 3, 6, and 9 fatty acids? What do they do for you? Fatty acids can be either saturated or unsaturated. Fatty acids are just one type of the macronutrient fat.

Omega 9. Omega 9s are unsaturated fatty acids commonly found in animal fat and vegetable oil. Two common Omega 9 fatty acids are oleic acid (the largest component of olive oil) and erucic acid, which is found in rapeseed (used in canola oil) and mustard seeds. Omega 9 is not an essential fatty acid, because the human body can make it. I do not recommend adding additional Omega 9 in a supplement. If you are eating enough olive oil, your body should be adequately supplied.

Omega 6. Omega 6 fatty acids are unsaturated fatty acids commonly found in poultry, eggs, avocados, nuts, soybean, rapeseed, and sunflower oil. There are several types of Omega 6 fatty acids, including linoleic acid (which is an essential fatty acid), gamma-linolenic acid, and arachidonic acid. Linoleic acid is the only essential Omega 6 fatty acid, because the human body cannot make it. Although our bodies need some linoleic acid to function properly, too much can cause inflammation throughout the body, leading to heart disease, asthma, and possibly even cancer. Most people do not need to take a supplement of Omega 6, because their diet should provide the right amount.

Omega 3. Omega 3 fatty acids are unsaturated fatty acids commonly found in fish oils, eggs, chicken, beef, and lamb, and to a lesser extent in olive oil and flaxseed oil. The three most well-known Omega 3 fatty acids are alpha linolenic acid (ALA), docosehexaenoic acid (DHA), and eicosapentaenoic acid (EPA). ALA is the essential Omega 3 fatty acid. DHA and EPA can both be produced to a limited extent by the body.

The Inuits and Omega 3. It was the eating habits and the lack of heart disease of Greenland's Inuit people that first shed light on the importance of Omega 3 fatty acids. This population consumes a large amount of fat from meat, but their rate of cardiovascular disease is very low. Supplementing with Omega 3 has been proposed to help with many different conditions, including heart disease, psychiatric disorders, cancer risk, immune function, arthritis, and asthma. For this reason, I recommend eating fish twice per week and also taking a daily supplement of Omega 3.

I learned my eating habits during what I call the "dark ages of nutrition" in the United States, when low-fat diets were all the rage. What did this trend do for us? According to the Harvard School of Public Health, in the 1960s, about 45 percent of the typical American diet was from fat. Only about 13 percent of the population was obese, and less than 1 percent had Type 2 diabetes. By lowering the fat in our diets to about 33 percent, we have increased the rate of obesity to almost 34 percent and Type 2 diabetes to 8 percent.

In our frenzy to cut all the fat out of our diet, we cut out the good fats as well. We then replaced these good fats, which have been proven to be heart healthy, with either trans fats, chemicals, or carbohydrates to make foods palatable. You can learn about the difference between fats that are good for you and fats that are not.

Have you ever heard of an essential carbohydrate? That's a trick question, because they don't exist! There are, however, such things as essential fatty acids and essential amino acids (building blocks of protein). They are called "essential" because the human body cannot make them—they have to be ingested. There are two essential fatty acids for humans: alpha-linolenic acid (an Omega 3 fatty acid) and linoleic acid (an Omega 6 fatty acid). Both of these fatty acids fall into the category of polyunsaturated fatty acids (PUFA).

Unsaturated Fatty Acids—The Good Kind of Fat

Both types of unsaturated fatty acids, MUFAs and PUFAs, are protective for heart disease. They raise your HDL cholesterol and lower your LDL. They are essential to proper functioning of your brain and nervous system. In the right proportion, they decrease inflammation throughout your body, decreasing atherosclerosis and improving asthma and arthritis. They improve your sense of satiety (feeling full), helping you to decrease your overall caloric intake and thus aid in weight loss.

Monounsaturated Fatty Acids (MUFAs)

Foods with high concentrations of MUFA include olive oil, canola oil, peanut oil, avocados, and most nuts and seeds. Remember that most foods have a complex makeup of various types of fatty acids, and are not purely one or the other. The Mediterranean diet has been studied extensively, particularly the diet of farmers on Crete, where the rate of heart disease is one of the lowest in the world. Some people in the Cretan study consumed almost one half-cup of olive oil per day. When we looked more closely into this phenomenon, it was discovered that two tablespoons per day is just as protective for heart disease as one half-cup. Table 3.1 shows the fat qualities of olive oil.

Table 3.1
Olive Oil Fatty Acid Components

Carbohydrate Options	Amount
Saturated fats	Up to 7 to 20%
Monounsaturated fats	Oleic acid: 55 to 83% (Omega 9 fatty acid)
Polyunsaturated fats	Linoleic acid: 3.5 to 21% (Omega 6 essential fatty acid) Alpha linolenic acid: < 1.5% (Omega 3 essential fatty acid)
Other good components in olive oil	Oleuropein or tyrosol, which are polyphenol antioxidants that lower the risk of cardiovascular disease

Two tablespoons of olive oil per day is a recommendation that always shocks my patients. Yes, I am aware that it is almost 240 calories, and that it is all fat. Some patients take a lot of convincing that the MUFAs/PUFAs that compose olive oil will not make them fat or raise their cholesterol. In fact, the fats in olive oil will improve your cholesterol numbers and lower your risk of cardiovascular disease. So how do you get that much olive oil into your diet? Use it throughout the day. Cook with it, because it is heat-stable and imparts a wonderful flavor to your food. Add it to your salads, even if you use another salad dressing. Pour it into a pita with vegetables, meat, falafel, and so on. Drizzle it over hummus for a snack with vegetables. I even pour a little on top of most of my soups.

Polyunsaturated Fatty Acids (PUFAs)

Polyunsaturated fatty acids (PUFAs) are the other type of unsaturated fatty acids. Brain cells are rich in some forms of PUFAs. Because of this fact, some research suggests that cognitive function (such as memory) is improved when PUFAs are made part of the diet. Research in maternal fetal medicine discovered this fact years ago, when manufacturers started to put DHA (a PUFA found in fish oil) in prenatal vitamins to improve IQ points in children. PUFAs also have an antiarrhythmic effect, aiding people with irregular heart rhythms to decrease or eliminate the medication they need to control this condition.

Sources of PUFA include soy, corn, sunflower, and flaxseed oils; fish; and walnuts. Omega 3 fatty acids are a PUFA found in the highest concentrations in fatty fish. Please eat fish at least two times per week to enhance your intake of Omega 3 fatty acids.

Saturated Fatty Acids

Our bodies can make all the saturated fat we need. Most meats, even the lean ones, have some saturated fat. The case against saturated fatty acids is not as clear as we once thought. When the studies that spawned the low-fat craze were scrutinized, some variables were found that cloud the picture. Most notable is the Oslo study done in the 1970s, a landmark study in the field of cardiology. It concluded that dietary fat caused ischemic heart disease. The problem is, that the men who were studied not only cut down on the saturated fat in their diet, but they also quit smoking. The control group continued to smoke. Thus it is difficult to say what caused the decrease in heart disease, the cessation of smoking or the lower saturated fat.

Although saturated fatty acids may not be as terrible for us as we once thought, the evidence is clear that substituting MUFA and PUFA is better when you can do so. Higher levels of MUFAs and PUFAs in our diet decrease the risk of coronary heart disease (CHD). Saturated fatty acids are not good for blood sugar regulation, but MUFAs and PUFAs are good for such regulation. Basically, substitute MUFAs and PUFAs when you can, but it is okay to have some saturated fat in your diet.

Some studies are looking into the effects of different saturated fatty acids. It may be that not all saturated fatty acids increase the risk of cardiovascular disease (CVD) to the same degree. There is no conclusive evidence at this point.

So what about butter? The take-home message about butter is to use it in moderation. When you can, substitute olive oil. Butter is mostly saturated fat, so use it sparingly. Yes, I know I just wrote that the verdict is still out on saturated fats; but we do know that MUFAs and PUFAs are good for you. So why not substitute them when you can?

Trans Fatty Acids

Trans fatty acids, or trans fats, are human-made fats created by heating liquid vegetable oils in the presence of hydrogen gas. This process, called hydrogenation, makes the oils more stable and less likely to spoil. They are used in the fast-food industry to fry food and to provide longer shelf-life for baked goods. Think about the baked goods that you make at home, and then compare that shelf-life to a snack that you get from a vending machine. Why does the homemade baked product break down and mold long before the vending-machine version? The answer is because the vending-machine version contains trans fats. Or how about that French fry that you find when cleaning your car, two months after you last ate fast food? A good rule of thumb is this: If nature can't break it down, maybe you should not eat it.

Fast-food restaurants are starting to get the message about the dangers of trans fats. The food that is now served at most restaurants is much lower in trans fat than it was ten years ago. This fact does not mean than fast food is now good for you. It is not! It is just slightly less harmful.

Manufacturers are now required to list how much trans fat is in a product on the label. This listing can be deceiving, because if there are 0.49 grams or less per serving, the manufacturer can list trans fat as 0. They may also list it as "hydrogenated" or "partially hydrogenated," which is the same thing as trans fat. So read food labels carefully! Trans fats lower your HDL (good cholesterol) and raise your LDL (bad cholesterol). Although there is an acceptable amount of saturated fat to have in your diet, there is no acceptable amount of trans fat. Trans fats have no nutritional value, and they can do nothing for you except cause harm by raising your blood cholesterol levels and increasing inflammation throughout your body.

The Best Ratio of Omega 6 to Omega 3 Is 4:1 or Less

Let's briefly review the best ratio of Omega 6 fatty acids to Omega 3 fatty acids in our modern diet. The typical U.S. diet has an Omega 6 to Omega 3 ratio of about 20:1. This ratio has a pro-inflammatory effect on the body. Any disease caused or made worse by inflammation, including heart disease, asthma, and arthritis, will be made worse by a high ratio.

The optimal ratio is 4:1 or less. We can shift this ratio by eating more fish, taking fish oil, eating free-range chicken and eggs, and consuming grass-fed beef. All of these foods have more Omega 3 fatty acids in them. Again, please don't look at this issue as "good versus bad." Omega 6 fatty acids are definitely good for us. One of the two essential fatty acids—linoleic acid—is an Omega 6. This program is about balance in the body. When you adjust your diet to improve the ratio between Omega 6 and Omega 3, you have gained another way to improve your overall health.

Cholesterol Test Results

These examples of lab reports show patients' cholesterol levels. The first test report is from someone who is following the Wellness 100 program. The second test report is from a different person who is not following Wellness 100. The person who is using the program is doing much better. Remember, these results are not from the same person, so obviously other factors come into account. But these examples will give you an idea what a good report looks like, in comparison to a not-so-good report.

Lipid Panel: Following the Program

Triglycerides	48 mg/dL
HDL cholesterol	61 mg/dL
VLDL cholesterol cal	10 mg/dL
LDL cholesterol calc	78 mg/dL
T. chol/HDL ratio	2.4 ratio units
Cholesterol, total	**149 mg/dL**

Lipid Panel: Not Following the Program

Cholesterol, total	**AB 227 mg/dL**
Triglycerides	AB 199 mg/dL
HDL cholesterol	42 mg/dL
VLDL cholesterol cal	40 mg/dL
LDL cholesterol calc	AB 145 mg/dL
T. chol/HDL ratio	AB 5.4 ratio units

High triglyceride levels reflect too many carbohydrates in the diet. They are a different type of lipid than cholesterol. Both cholesterol and triglycerides are transported in your bloodstream by little spheres covered in protein; these spheres are called lipoproteins.

HDL: This means high-density lipoprotein, or "good" cholesterol.

LDL: This means low-density lipoprotein, which is considered "bad" cholesterol. When elevated, LDL increases the risk for heart disease.

VLDL: This means very low-density lipoprotein, which contains cholesterol, protein, and triglycerides. It contains high levels of triglycerides, and it is calculated as a percentage of your triglycerides. When elevated, VLDL increases the risk for heart disease.

Ratio: A ratio of less than 5:1 is recommended by the American Heart Association.

Total cholesterol: The total cholesterol number will be more than the HDL and the LDL added together, because there are more lipoproteins to be counted.

Cholesterol

What is cholesterol, if it is not a fatty acid? This is a hard question to answer, and it requires a small chemistry lesson. Cholesterol is a waxy, breakdown product of an organic compound. It can be found in the cell membranes and plasma of all animals. Cholesterol is recycled in the liver and is excreted into the digestive tract. About 50 percent of it is then reabsorbed by the small intestine. Dietary sources of cholesterol include cheese, eggs, beef, pork, poultry, and shrimp. It can be found in plant sources as well, but usually to a lesser extent. Many plants contain a cholesterol-like substance called phytosterols, which have been shown to lower cholesterol.

We need cholesterol. Our bodies make cholesterol in higher quantities than we absorb from food. Without cholesterol, we cannot make a lot of the substances vital to our health. I am reminded of this fact by a female patient I worked with when I was straight out of my residency. This patient came to my office saying that she was not having periods. She looked healthy and was in her late twenties, but she had a bizarre lipid panel. She followed no specific diet, and she ate whatever she wanted. Her total cholesterol level was below 80. Cholesterol is the substance from which all of our hormones are made. When we don't have enough cholesterol, we can't make our estrogens, progesterone, testosterone, and so on that we need in sufficient quantities. In the case of this patient, insufficient hormones led to her not having periods. Unfortunately, I don't think this patient believed me when I told her that her very low cholesterol was a bad thing.

Most evidence is now associating only a small increase in our blood cholesterol levels with the cholesterol that we consume. The real dangers to our cholesterol (both in the type and amount of LDL cholesterol) are trans fats and carbohydrates. We are discovering that not all LDL cholesterol is created equal. Certain types of "bad" cholesterol are worse for us than others. Almost 50 percent of heart attack victims have normal cholesterol numbers. Obviously, we are missing something. Is cholesterol found at the scene of the crime but not guilty, or is there more to the story? This section should clarify the cholesterol mystery.

High-Density and Low-Density Lipoproteins

What exactly are HDL and LDL, and all the other letters that you see on your lab report? Cholesterol is not a ball of fat floating around in your bloodstream. It is contained in little protein-covered spheres called lipoproteins. HDL are high-density lipoproteins, and LDL are low-density lipoproteins. High-density lipoproteins are considered to be our good cholesterol. Their job in the body is to help remove triglycerides from the bloodstream and take them back to the liver for disposal. Having high HDL lowers your risk for heart disease.

The job of LDL is to carry cholesterol from the liver to other parts of the body. Certain cells in our body then extract the fat and cholesterol from the LDL molecule to be used for various functions. We now know that LDL comes in many shapes and sizes. We even know which of these are worse for you. When we examine LDL cholesterol more closely, we can see that some particles are large and buoyant, and others are small and dense. When the majority of your LDL is the small, dense type, you have a higher

LDL-P, or particle number. This high LDL-P will increase your risk for heart disease threefold, because the small, dense particles are better able to get into the walls of your arteries. They are also more susceptible to oxidation from free radicals. Oxidized LDL then enters cells called macrophages (found in the lining of our arteries), to form cholesterol-rich plaques. It is these plaques that cause narrowing of the arteries and, when the plaques rupture, cause heart attacks or strokes.

We usually see a higher LDL particle number (meaning more of the small, dense type) associated with a higher triglyceride level. Both of these are caused by a diet high in carbohydrates. When you eat too many carbohydrates, not only does the increase in insulin lead to more production of cholesterol by your liver, but also the type of cholesterol that is much worse for you.

Embrace Eggs

For years I avoided eating eggs, because I was terrified that they were bad for me. This avoidance is also the biggest dietary "brag" I get from my patients. I ask all patients at their annual visit about their diet. Most of my patients are very health conscious, and they try to do the right things with their nutrition. They almost always tell me that they never fry anything, eat lots of fiber-rich foods and fruits, and only use egg substitutes. They look at me as if I have lost my mind when I tell them to eat eggs. Eggs are the richest source of cholesterol in a westernized diet. Following this advice of mine will raise one's cholesterol and cause heart disease, right?

Not exactly.

Studies have demonstrated that the cholesterol we eat has only a modest effect, if any, on our blood cholesterol levels. About 20 percent of people are hyper-responders to dietary cholesterol, and it will raise their cholesterol by about 5 percent. Even in the group of hyper-responders, the effect on cholesterol is to increase the LDL but lower the particle number. So it makes more of the "good type of bad cholesterol," the type that does not increase the risk of heart disease. Furthermore, even the modest increase was seen only with a larger amount of eggs than most people eat per day—three eggs or more. Several studies found no increase in cholesterol when egg consumption was coupled with weight loss. This is why thirty years of research has failed to prove that cholesterol from eggs increases cardiovascular disease. So forget what you have been taught about eggs and embrace them as a wonderful source of protein.

Eggs are also an excellent source of vitamins C, E, and B12, as well as folate. They have high levels of lutein and zeaxanthin, which prevent age-related diseases such as Alzheimer's and macular degeneration. They are an energy-dense food and will not leave you feeling hungry, as typical high-carbohydrate breakfasts do. They also are a portable source of protein. Try hard-boiling eggs the night before and keeping them in your refrigerator. You can then grab them in the morning to eat at your desk for breakfast or to add protein to a salad for lunch.

Eggs contain eighteen different vitamins and minerals. One large egg has 0.36 grams of carbohydrates, 1.6 grams of saturated fat, 1.8 grams of monounsaturated fat, and 1 gram of polyunsaturated fat, with 6.3 grams of protein.

What to Remember: MUFAs and PUFAs Are Essential, But Trans Fats Are Bad

The most important thing to remember from this chapter is this: Monounsaturated fatty acids (MUFAs) and polyunsaturated fatty acids (PUFAs) are good for you. They do not make you fat. MUFAs and PUFAs are essential for your body to function normally. They raise your good cholesterol, lower your bad cholesterol, and decrease your risk for cardiovascular disease. Saturated fatty acids should be eaten in moderation; substitute with MUFAs and PUFAs when you can. Never eat trans fatty acids. (Please read this paragraph a couple more times!)

CHAPTER 4

The Power of Protein

We have discussed carbohydrates and fats, and we can now move on to macronutrient number three: protein. What fears do we have about protein? Most anti-protein sentiment comes from the fat that is often found with protein in nature. Many of my patients proudly tell me that they have given up meat. But vegetarians must be careful to find other sources of protein. There is nothing dangerous in lean meats (except antibiotics and hormones, if the meat is not organic). Remember from the fats chapter (which you just read) that there is an acceptable amount of saturated fat that we can eat, which translates to an acceptable amount of fat in our meats. Just as there are essential fatty acids, there are essential amino acids. These essential amino acids are the building blocks of protein, without which the body cannot function properly. In this chapter you will learn about essential amino acids. You'll realize why I suggest a minimum of 70 grams of protein per day, and you will find out about the best sources of these proteins.

Points to Remember about Protein

- *Minimum of 70 grams per day*
  If only from meat sources, this amount translates to about 9 ounces of meat per day.
- *Maximum of 10 grams of protein from dairy*
  Dairy is okay in moderation; but if you have yogurt for breakfast, that is your entire dairy for the day.
- *Choose lean meats only*
  Lean meats have less saturated fat.
- *Choose grass-fed meats when available*
  Grass-fed meats have a better ratio of Omega 6 to Omega 3.
- *Choose organic when possible*
- *Add protein when you can*
  Try protein powder in your smoothies.
  Add tuna, ham, or eggs to salads.
  Drop an egg in your stir-fry.
  Save leftover meat from dinner to add to breakfast.

Recommended Daily Amount

A popular misconception when starting a high-protein diet is that it is "all or nothing" (meaning all protein and no carbohydrates). Extremes in our diet do not work. I have tried them all—low fat; no carbohydrate; and extremely low calorie. After a few weeks, like most people, I always quit. Balance does work, and Wellness 100 seeks balance based on good science. When high-protein diets are studied, the numbers are not as drastic as you might assume. Most studies used 30 percent of total calories, or a range between 60 to 120 grams of protein per day. Other studies considered a ratio between carbohydrates and protein of 1:1.

I remember the first time that I ate a low-carbohydrate diet! I spent an entire month eating beef jerky and eggs, with pickles as my snack. I followed the rules of the diet, but I did not really understand the big picture. Our low-carbohydrate program still recommends more carbohydrates daily than protein. Think about that recommendation; I want you to get 100 grams of carbohydrates daily and a minimum of 70 grams of protein. Obviously, there is room for more protein, depending on the good fats you consume.

Satiety (Feeling Full)

Before I learned better, one of my biggest arguments against breakfast was that it made me hungry the rest of the day. Have you ever noticed that happening to you? Traditional breakfast foods are high in carbohydrates, and they don't "stick with you" like protein. Proteins, unlike carbohydrates, cause an increased feeling of satiety or fullness. Numerous research articles have proven this fact. If you want more proof, however, try your own experiment. Try the typical cereal, juice, and fruit breakfast one morning; then, the next day, eat a balanced breakfast with 30 grams of carbohydrates and the appropriate amount of fat and protein. When you aren't snacking by 10 a.m., you will have your proof!

My patients are always amazed, when starting Wellness 100, that despite lowering their daily calories, they are not hungry. Why is this? The increased sensation of fullness or satiety with a higher-protein diet may be caused by specific hormones that are released from the body. Some research suggests that we feel full because of the protein's thermogenic (heat-producing) effect. (This effect is discussed next.) Furthermore, it appears that protein from animal sources is more filling than protein from plant sources. Whatever the reason, feeling full will have the added benefit of helping you eat less.

Thermogenic Effect

All foods are thermogenic, because the body must burn calories to digest them. Fat has the lowest thermogenic effect, and protein has the highest. The best thermogenic foods are lean meats, seafood, and eggs. So when you eat these foods, you are burning more calories just to process them. This process is called thermogenesis.

Weight Maintenance

We have studied weight loss for a long time, but what do we know about maintaining our desired weight? A popular diet right now is the hcg diet. I don't recommend this diet to my patients, because I don't recommend crash dieting. Anyone will lose weight on 500 to 800 calories per day, but you won't learn any good habits to help you keep it off. You will notice that the title of this book does not even contain the word diet. When people think about going on a diet, they expect to do it for a few weeks or months until they reach their goal, then go back to eating "normally." Wellness 100 should become your normal. Studies are now showing that higher-protein diets are more effective at maintaining weight loss than high-carbohydrate diets. You will discover that when you achieve your weight-loss goal, it is very easy to continue to count your 100 carbohydrates and let the fat and protein fall into place. You may no longer need to count the calories to maintain your weight.

Bone and Muscle Maintenance

Researchers are now finding out how important protein is to our bones and muscle mass, especially as we age. Osteoporosis (a loss of bone mass) and sarcopenia (a loss of muscle mass) are important risk factors for many diseases of aging. Detractors of high-protein diets warn that such diets can damage your kidneys. However, someone with normal kidney function can easily process up to 1.4 grams of protein per kilogram (kg) of body weight safely. That means that a 120-pound person can consume more than 70 grams of protein per day. That is why we have proposed 70 grams of protein as a minimum daily. As you lose weight, keeping the protein high in your diet should prevent the loss of muscle or bone mass.

Body Composition

Even if you lose the same amount of weight with a high-carbohydrate versus a high-protein diet, you will be happier with the results of the high-protein diet. Carbohydrates put weight around the body's middle. When you eat a higher-protein diet, you lose weight in the gut. Beer bellies are carbohydrate bellies! Traditionally, "apples" (people with most of their weight around the middle) have a higher risk of heart disease than "pears," those of us with bigger hips.

Essential Amino Acids

Essential amino acids, like essential fatty acids, cannot be made by the body and must be ingested. There are nine essential amino acids for adults, and an additional three that are considered essential for children. Some of the things that these amino acids do for you are the following: bone development and collagen formation, nerve function, formation of red blood cells, regulating blood sugar and energy levels, help with sleep and anxiety, and the formation of tooth enamel. See Table 4.1 to learn about essential amino acids.

Table 4.1

Essential Amino Acids

Essential Amino Acids for Adults	Where They Are Found	Importance in the Human Body
Isoleucine	Eggs, soy, poultry, cheese, fish, lamb	Build and maintain muscle mass
Leucine	Soy, beef, pork, fish, almonds, peanuts, chicken, eggs	Build and maintain muscle mass
Lysine	Catfish, chicken, beef, soy, cheese, lentils, eggs, milk	Used to make collagen
Methionine	Eggs, Brazil nuts, sesame seeds, chicken, fish, peanuts, lentils	Methyl donor, and important to the body's natural detoxification system
Phenylalanine	Eggs, soy, peanuts, fish, cheese	Important for brain function and mood
Threonine	Poultry, fish, cottage cheese, meat, lentils	Formation of collagen and elastin in the skin
Tryptophan	Eggs, soy, fish, pumpkin seeds, cheese, turkey, pork, chicken, beef, salmon, lamb	Used to make serotonin (helps with depression) and melatonin (helps with sleep)
Valine	Soy, eggs, cheese, sesame seeds, fish	Build and maintain muscle
Histidine	Soy, eggs, cheese, fish, venison, beef	Important for the immune system and blood cell production

Essential Amino Acids for Children	Where They Are Found	Importance in the Human Body
Cysteine	Pork, poultry, eggs, dairy, garlic, onions, broccoli, wheat germ	Help the liver with detoxification; converted into a powerful antioxidant
Arginine	Dairy, beef, pork, fish, poultry, wild game	Help with wound healing and immune function
Tyrosine	Soy, poultry, fish, almonds, peanuts, avocados, dairy	Important for a properly functioning neurologic system

Sources of Protein

Meat as a Source of Protein

Do not be afraid to eat meat. Even red meat is healthy, when consumed in moderation and when you chose the leanest cuts. Lean meats are high in nutrients such as zinc, vitamin B12, selenium, phosphorus, niacin, vitamin B6, riboflavin, and iron. Meat contains all of the essential amino acids. Remember, these are the building blocks of protein necessary to your body to keep you healthy. The fat content of meat depends on the type of meat, as well as how the animal was fed.

I grew up on a cattle farm. I know how most cows are fed. On the farm, they eat grass and hay. This diet produces leaner beef with a better ratio of Omega 6 to Omega 3. However, most calves become feeder calves. They are sold off to feedlots, where they are slaughtered before they are two years old. In order to encourage growth and profits for the company, they are fed grain, protein supplements, growth hormones, and (when necessary) antibiotics. Obviously, grass-fed beef is the better choice. You will get more Omega 3 fatty acids, and you will avoid the antibiotics and growth hormones found in the more commercially available beef. The same goes for chicken, and even the eggs that the hens lay. Always buy free-range, grass-fed chicken and eggs.

One nutrient found almost exclusively in red meat is carnitine. In the body, it helps convert fat to energy. Low carnitine levels may cause fatigue and aging signs in the skin, specifically wrinkles. It is a powerful antioxidant. There is promising evidence for the use of carnitine as a supplement for treating and preventing heart disease and irregular heart rhythms. Because carnitine is not found in any great amount in grains, fruits, or vegetables, if you are a vegetarian, you should take carnitine as a supplement. Appendix B contains nutritional information for beef, poultry, pork, and so forth.

Vegetarian Sources of Protein

I am not anti-vegetarian. However, I do believe that eating meat will make it easier for you to get the right amount of protein. If you are a vegetarian, you have to be proactive in getting enough protein. You may need to use protein powders. Concentrate on legumes, grains, and vegetables with a higher amount of protein. Appendix B contains information to help you do this.

The Case Against Casein

Casein is the name of a group of proteins found in dairy. In fact, there are four casein proteins that make up 80 percent of the protein in cows' milk. T. Collin Campbell's *The China Study* (2006) suggests a correlation between powdered, isolated casein fed to rats and the promotion of cancer-cell growth when exposed to carcinogens (known cancer-causing substances). Campbell's research started in China, where people in certain provinces have virtually no cancer. In recording their diets, he discovered that they eat very little animal protein. He then went to the lab to determine whether there was a cause-and-effect relationship between protein from animal sources and cancer. Campbell studied casein and its ability to cause cancer; and he did, in fact, conclude that there was a relationship. Controversy, however, surrounds his conclusions from the study. Campbell concluded (in very broad generalizations) that all animal proteins are dangerous. However, other studies suggest (as when you look closely at Campbell's research) a dose-dependent cancer risk for casein. I think there is enough evidence to suggest moderation in dairy consumption. The risk seems to be dose-dependent, and fewer than 10 grams of casein per day seems to be relatively safe.

Remember, this program seeks to take the best scientific research and blend it together to find the best eating habits. It would be naïve to think that one culture has it completely right when it comes to diet and health. If, for instance, we took Campbell's initial findings and cut all animal protein out of our diet, we would be missing out on a lot of essential amino acids, vital minerals, and vitamins. Remember carnitine? If you eat no red meat (no carnitine), you will start to look and feel older. Programs that preach absolutes when it comes to diet will always leave you lacking in something that your body needs.

Fish

Eating fish is an excellent way to get more Omega 3 fatty acids in your diet. Omega 3s are important for your brain, heart, and joints, just to name a few of the benefits. As with any food, there are better choices that can be made within this category.

One of my favorite eating disaster stories came from Larry, a co-worker of my husband's. Larry had come to work at noon one day with a bag of fried, fast-food fish. He had just been to the doctor's office, where he was told that he had high cholesterol, that he should eat healthier, and that he should get more fish in his diet. Hush puppies are not fish! Fried fish negates any of the health benefits that you may have gotten from the fish. Many fast-food fish restaurants now have baked and broiled choices, so if you really like these restaurants, you now have better choices.

When choosing fish to prepare at home or when choosing from a menu at a restaurant, avoid shark, swordfish, king mackerel, ocean perch, striped bass, or tilefish. They contain high levels of mercury. As a rule of thumb, the longer a fish lives and the higher on the food chain it is, it will contain higher levels of mercury. Never eat the skin, because any toxin found in fish will be concentrated in the skin.

Buy wild-caught seafood, when available. The floating nets and pens used for farm-raised fish can trap pollutants and bacteria, making it necessary to use antibiotics and herbicides. Never buy farm-raised salmon. Farm-raised salmon is not naturally pink, like the wild-caught variety. Because the grey/white color of this fish is not appealing to consumers, farmers may use dye to make the fish look like the characteristic pink color.

Choose saltwater over freshwater fish when you can. Contaminants in our rivers and lakes are more concentrated than in the ocean. Even when eating out, you can usually learn the source of the fish if you ask.

As with everything in Wellness 100, this chapter is a tool to help you make the best choices. I would rather you eat fish, even if it is farm raised, than not eat fish at all. The health benefits still outweigh the risks.

Health Benefits of High-Protein Diets

One example of the health benefits of protein can be found in the Nurses' Health Study. The group of women in the study who had the lowest risk of cardiovascular disease had the highest protein intake (24 percent of calories). This result may be due to the lowering of triglycerides seen when protein is substituted for carbohydrates. It could also be because of the improvement in the LDL particle number. Remember, LDL cholesterol is your bad cholesterol, but not all bad cholesterol is created equal. It can be found in big, fluffy balls or little, harmful balls; both are floating in your bloodstream. The smaller the balls of LDL, the higher your particle number, and the more risk you have of cardiovascular disease. High-protein diets (30 percent of calories) also have also been shown to provide improved glucose control in people with Type 2 diabetes.

Wellness 100 has a favorable balance between carbohydrates and protein that will help you lose weight, especially around the middle. It will help you maintain lean muscle mass while losing weight. You will improve your overall health and decrease your risk for heart attack, stroke, and diabetes. You also will retain a youthful appearance longer. What more could you want from your diet? All of this can be done without eating the same boring things every day, as the second part of this book will teach you.

So remember, choose sources of protein that have more MUFA and PUFA and less saturated fats. These sources will be nuts, seeds, and lean meats. Beans are also a good source of protein; but if you try to get all your protein from beans, you will probably be consuming too many carbohydrates. Seventy (70) grams of protein per day is the minimum that you should include in your diet.

CHAPTER 5
Eating Out

Eating meals at home helps you to stay on any diet. But eating every meal at home is not realistic for most of us. In this chapter you will find helpful tips on planning ahead for workday meals and survival tips for eating out.

Breakfast

The best advice for eating out for breakfast is: don't! Make your best effort to eat breakfast at home or at least to make breakfast and take it with you. If you have to get up five or ten minutes earlier to make breakfast, then that is what you need to do. You won't get any sympathy from me on this issue. I have been an obstetrician for about ten years, and even with the unpredictability of my schedule, I still manage to eat breakfast at home most mornings. It only takes me seven minutes to make a breakfast sandwich. If I am in a hurry, I wrap it in foil and eat it on the way to work. If I know I have an early-morning meeting, I fix a smoothie the night before and put it in the blender in the morning, pour it into a to-go cup, and go.

If you are on vacation or just feel like going out for breakfast, choose a sit-down restaurant. This way, you can make choices such as a piece of lean meat, egg, whole wheat toast, oatmeal, or whatever you can find on the menu that will fit into the program. Breakfast menus are really geared to this program, because most give you so many choices and combinations. Breakfast is especially dangerous for overdoing it on carbohydrates, because it is easy and cheap to pull through a fast-food line or get pastries. But if you avoid the drive-through pitfalls, getting a balanced breakfast at a sit-down restaurant is easy. The one caution on this—be careful about your portions, and know how many eggs, pieces of toast, fruit, or meat you can fit into your meal in advance.

Lunch

Whenever possible, take your lunch to work. When you must eat out, make better choices. As always, avoid fast foods. If fast food is your only option, go as plain as you can. Get a salad when you can, and use your own olive oil. Order the snack size or kid's portions, if available. Try wraps instead of buns. Order grilled instead of fried, and stay away from the french fries. Tacos are not a bad option; but again, order as plain as you can. Heavy portions of sour cream, cheese, and so forth just add unwanted calories.

Be aware of the calories in your beverages. Order water with your lunch. Sweet tea, sodas, energy drinks, and what I refer to as "frou-frou coffees" are loaded with sugary calories.

Avoid getting stuck and desperate. You should be hungry at lunch, but not so starved that you eat the first thing you can get your hands on. Keep nuts or other healthy snack options at work so that you have the patience to make a good lunch choice.

Dinner

Eating dinner out should be a treat. It should be about socializing or celebrating, rather than a way of life.

I had one patient who had a very hard time with this part of the program. She and her husband both worked full time, and their children were grown. Neither of them enjoyed cooking, so they ate out every night. She did well for several weeks on the program, and she even lost weight while still eating out once or twice per week. But eventually she went back to her old habit of eating out every night and gained it all back. You will never be able to maintain a healthy lifestyle if you eat out a lot. Once a week, or less, is optimal for eating dinner out. Anything you can eat out, you can make at home with a lot fewer calories. So on those occasions when you do eat out, here are some tips to make "dinner out" work with the program.

Do some research. If you are going to a chain restaurant, pull up their website before you go. Almost all restaurants have their nutrition information on the internet. This way, you can pick the dinner that appeals to you and that fits the program. As always, don't forget to factor in beverages.

Try not to turn chips and salsa into the "meal before the meal." Yes, they taste yummy with lots of salt, but either push them to the side, or ask that they not be brought to your table. Learn to say no to these freebies and others, like crispy noodles at Chinese restaurants, or baskets of bread and muffins.

Eat a salad before the meal. Watery foods like lettuce have been shown to make you feel fuller. This is also a great way to include raw vegetables in your meal. Be careful with dressings. Try ordering just olive oil instead. If you must have dressing, order it on the side, and dip your salad into it—you will use less dressing with this method. This rule holds true for all sauces and condiments. You may feel a bit high-maintenance when you order, but what's the harm? You have to watch out for your health.

Portions at restaurants are usually too large. Try ordering a side salad and splitting an entrée. This amount will come much closer to being the right amount of food. Pick an entrée that is not based on pasta. Gravitate toward a meal complete with enough protein, vegetables, and a small amount of carbohydrates. If no one will split a meal with you, remember that you can always get a doggie bag! Still order the salad; but when your meal comes, portion it out more reasonably. Cut your meat in half. Push the carbs to the side, except for maybe a bite or two, and eat all of your vegetables. Better yet, ask to substitute another helping of vegetables for your carbohydrate side.

Avoid buffets. The temptation is too great to eat too much. You will eat fast and fill your plate with a lot of food. Buffets are of no value if they destroy your health.

Get into a habit of frequenting your favorite restaurants and knowing what you can eat. For instance, my husband and I love Mexican food. We could eat it every day, and we make it at home several times per week. We meet about once per week at our favorite place in town for lunch. Most of the time, I am successful at pushing the chips away. We then order fajitas and split them, and I don't use any of the tortillas. I eat about half the beans and none of the rice. This method fits the program very well, and because we are having lunch, I am not even tempted by the margarita!

Which brings us again to the issue of beverages and having fun when eating out. Don't drink your calories. It is so much more satisfying, especially at a restaurant, to eat them instead. The calories in all kinds of drinks add up too fast. Drinks just aren't worth it.

A few last points for eating out—or eating at home, for that matter. First, eat in courses. Have a salad first, then eat your meal. Don't have the plates all come out together. This tactic will slow you down and allow your brain to register what your stomach is telling it. It takes 20 minutes for your brain to get the signals from your stomach that you are full. When was the last time you took more than 20 minutes to eat a meal? Second, set your fork down between bites. This method will slow you down. Remember to drink water during a meal. Water takes up space in your stomach. Last, try chewing your food thirty times before you swallow. This age-old advice really does work.

Dining at Someone's House

There are times when you just have to smile and eat whatever is served. You may be at an important dinner and don't want to give offense. Or perhaps your grandmother made your favorite cookies. Generally speaking, though when you are dining with people who will understand (good friends or family), it is not rude to eat healthy even if no one else does.

If it is a potluck, bring a vegetable tray with a healthy dip, or a large salad filled with good protein. You can then fill your caloric needs without having to try to find the "least of the evils" of whatever else is served. If the meal at someone's house is not a potluck, you can still ask your host if you can bring something. If your host has provided everything, you will have to make some choices.

My Grandmother Marie was not a small woman. At family functions, she would always say that she had not eaten all day so that she could eat whatever she wanted that night. Don't do this! Eat normally during the day, even if you have a function to go to that evening. You may save up some of your calories for the evening, but try to be reasonable. Try 20 percent of your calories for breakfast and 20 percent for lunch, leaving you more to play with for dinner. But remember, you cannot save up your carbohydrates. Say no to dessert or politely take just a few bites.

At big parties, especially around holidays and the Super Bowl, you can be bombarded with horrible "party food," including chips and dips, pizza, hot dogs, and dessert. You may need to eat before you go or when you get home. Plan your day so that you are full when you get there and not tempted to eat junk.

Summer parties can be especially dangerous. Most BBQ sauce is loaded with sugar. When you are served sugar-coated meat, potato salad, and gooey desserts, it is hard to make good choices. (When you're the host, use a dry rub on your meat instead of BBQ sauce.) Gravitate toward the cole slaw instead of the potato salad, and try to resist the desserts. You can find things, even at a BBQ, that will fit into the program.

I know there are times to forget the program and enjoy. Birthdays are one. (Your birthday, not every one of your 100 closest friends' birthdays.) Holidays (*the* holiday) and anniversaries, as well as other big occasions, should be counted outside of everyday life. Life is too short not to let loose every once in a while. Make those occasions special, enjoy the "splurge," and resume your Wellness 100 eating habits. You'll do just fine.

CHAPTER 6
Hidden Calories and Hidden Dangers

As you learned in previous chapters, it is not just how much you eat, but what you eat that affects your health and weight. You cannot live on beef jerky and think that you are getting proper protein. Likewise, all of your carbohydrates cannot be from soda. In this chapter, you will learn more about how to make wise food and drink choices. This chapter will discuss the empty calories in most beverages; the harmful effects of additives, preservatives, and artificial sweeteners; and the hidden dangers of dairy. You will get the cutting-edge news on the emerging study of obesogens (chemical compounds that make you fat) and find out about the dangers of plastics.

Beverages

A patient recently complained to me that she could not lose weight. A review of her diet showed she drank two, 2-liter bottles of soda per day. (I am not making this up!) Many people today have no idea how many calories they consume in beverages. A 2007 analysis of U.S. beverage trends revealed that about 25 percent of our average calorie consumption is from liquids. Perhaps you like to drink an occasional margarita. Well, you may as well have a Big Mac; the two have about the same calories. That sad situation holds true for most mixed drinks.

Calories from beverages are not as filling for several reasons. The biggest reason is that beverages are almost all carbohydrates. What is the number one rule of Wellness 100? Never consume carbohydrates alone; they cause weight gain around the middle and make you hungry. So when you reach for a thirst-quenching soda, sweet tea, or energy drink, it is only going to make you more hungry an hour or so later. Remember the temporary boost in serotonin that you get from carbohydrates and caffeine? Consuming beverages containing one or both of those will make your body crave another boost of serotonin. To avoid a serotonin crash, you will be drawn to something sugary or caffeinated, which will only perpetuate the cycle. This fact is why people don't lose weight on diet soda.

Another reason not to drink your calories is that the glycemic index in drinks is much higher than in other foods. This situation is obvious when you think of the sweeteners in soft drinks, such as sugar and high fructose corn syrup. But please remember that this fact holds true for juices as well. Fruit juice contains good vitamins and minerals from the fruit, but none of the fiber. Without the fiber, the glycemic index goes up, your blood sugars go up faster, and your insulin levels shoot up. Insulin is very damaging to the lining of blood vessels; so for our longevity, this damaging process is something we want to avoid.

Finally, because beverages are in liquid form already and have a high glycemic index, your body does not have to expend a lot of energy breaking them down. Energy expenditure equals calories lost. So you will want to consume fewer calories than your body uses, in order to lose weight. In Table 6.1, you will find some examples of beverages and their calories and carbohydrates. When you have the choice between drinking your calories and being able to consume more calories in actual food, I hope you can see that food is not only more satisfying but also better for you.

A word on juicing. I have a lot of patients who love to juice, and they throw a lot of fruits and veggies into a juicer for breakfast. This practice is okay, as long as you also keep the fiber component and drink the fiber down with the juice. Also, a glass of juice is mostly carbohydrates, so you need either to eat some protein with it or add a protein powder.

Alcohol

How many times have you heard the warning, "Consume alcohol in moderation"? It's good advice. If you want to have a glass of wine because it complements a meal, that is fine. You must count it into your calories and carbohydrates. Alcohol is in its own class for calorie calculation. One gram of pure alcohol contains seven calories. If the alcohol has any sugar in it, as does wine (not even added sugar, just the natural sugar), then you have to add in the calories from the carbohydrates. Essentially, a 4-ounce glass of red wine has about 100 calories and 4.4 grams of carbohydrates. See how quickly that could add up if you are not careful? I find a useful tip is to set aside those big wine glasses and use a small tumbler or a cordial glass for a glass of wine. You won't be tempted to pour as much.

Table 6.1
Common Beverages and Their Nutritional Values

Beverage in Ounces	Calories*	Carbohydrates in Grams*
Cola, 12 ounces	143	40 grams
Red wine, 4 ounces	102	4.4 grams
White wine, 4 ounces	96	4.4 grams
Margarita, 8 ounces	300 to 400+	30 to 70 grams, depending on how sweet
Long Island iced tea, 8 ounces	270	33 grams
Apple juice, 4 ounces	59	14.3 grams
Grape juice, 4 ounces	85	22 grams
Orange juice, 4 ounces	54	12.8 grams
Sweet tea, 4 ounces	35+	8.6+ grams, depending on how sweet
Energy drink, 8.5-ounce can	113+	28.2+ grams, depending on brand
Latte, 8 ounces (plain)	67	10 grams
Beer, 12 ounces	145	10.6 grams

*Amounts are averages, and individual calories and carbohydrates will vary.

Food Additives

About 2,500 chemicals can be considered "food additives." I am not going to address all of them, but the following information will give you an idea of what some of the most common additives are, and what they can do to you. In general, it is best to avoid as many additives as possible. Avoid packaged foods, eat fresh fruits and vegetables and lean organic meats, and this issue of additives won't be a problem for you.

The U.S. Food and Drug Administration (FDA) studies all additives closely to determine any toxicity to humans. An acceptable daily intake (ADI) of additives is then established. The ADI is a calculation that assumes that there is an acceptable risk that people are willing to take from this chemical, so that they can eat the foods that they want. Food in its natural state, like broccoli, does not have an ADI. I find the ADI to be a scary concept. If we consume these products, we are damaging our system. But apparently the nation is willing to accept the risk, so that we can eat things we shouldn't eat in the first place.

Nitrites

Nitrate and nitrite salts of sodium and potassium are used as preservatives for foods such as meats, cheeses, and pickled herring. These chemical compounds can combine with chemicals in the stomach to make nitrosamine, which is a carcinogen (a cancer-causing agent). Whenever possible, look for labels on meats and cheeses that say "nitrite/nitrate free." Bacon is notorious for containing these nitrites. If you do choose to consume these preservatives, then having vitamin C in your diet may help protect your body from the negative effects of nitrites.

Artificial Sweeteners

Aspartame. The acceptable daily intake of aspartame set by the FDA is 50 mg/kg of body weight. Natural sweeteners like honey and agave don't have a limit set by the FDA. If aspartame is not harmful, why is there an acceptable daily limit?

Aspartame is metabolized in our gut to its three metabolites: aspartic acid, phenylalanine, and methanol. When methanol is further broken down in our systems, it becomes formaldehyde. Formaldehyde is commonly known as "embalming fluid." It is important to note that many natural foods, especially fruit juices, also have formaldehyde as a breakdown product. But when found in nature, this product is always with ethanol, which is the natural antidote to methanol and formaldehyde.

Many people are allergic to aspartame. This problem is not the anaphylactic (throat swelling) type of allergy, but a milder form. It can cause headaches, nausea, or fatigue for some people, and even seizures. But maybe some people think that it's worth a little headache to use this artificial sweetener? If the minor side effects don't scare you, the next side effects will.

Aspartame has been linked to several different types of cancer. Many reliable studies on rats have demonstrated increased rates of lymphomas and leukemias. There seems even to be a risk to a growing fetus if a pregnant woman consumes aspartame. Aspartame may also damage our nervous system and cause behavioral changes.

Splenda. We don't yet have a lot of good data out there on Splenda. It is an artificial sweetener made with sucralose and the fillers maltodextrin and glucose. What we do know so far is that it alters good bacteria in your gut. When this change happens, it can cause loose stools or constipation. Other side effects are a decrease in immune function, as well as food sensitivities and allergies. Seventy percent of your immune system is in your gut, so when you disturb its delicate balance, there are far-reaching effects. This altering process can also diminish the effectiveness of oral medications.

If you want something sweet, just eat something sweet. If you need to drink something sweet, you are better off with regular soda than the diet variety. Artificial sweeteners like aspartame have no redeeming qualities. It is best to cut them completely out of your diet!

High Fructose Corn Syrup. Since the early 1980s, high fructose corn syrup (HFCS) has been substituted as a sweetener in an ever-increasing number of beverages, condiments, breakfast cereals, and snack foods. It is cheaper than table sugar, and it is an easy ingredient to use because it mixes well with most foods.

HFCS is a hot topic in current food research. Although it has the same amount of calories per gram as pure cane sugar (table sugar), the chemical composition of HFCS is different. Regular sugar is 50 percent fructose and 50 percent glucose. HFCS varies in its composition, but it can range from 55–80 percent fructose and the remainder glucose. So what is the problem with HFCSs? Glucose, fructose—they are both sugar, so does it really matter how we get our sugar calories? In contrast to glucose, fructose gets broken down by the liver more quickly and leads to more of a rise in triglycerides and fat storage. Some researchers suggest that the feeling of fullness or satiety in response to insulin release and leptin do not occur as readily with HFCS as they do with table sugar. This situation could lead to an increase in consumption and partially account for the increased weight gain seen with HFCS.

A 2010 Princeton study showed that when rats fed a diet of HFCS were compared with rats fed table sugar in the same amounts, the HFCS rats gained more weight. The weight distribution was more in the abdomen than in other regions of the body. Triglyceride levels also increased.

As I have mentioned before, some truths are hard for me to publish. My father is a farmer who raised cattle and grows corn. Having said that, I think there is enough research to prove that high fructose corn syrup is worse for you than other sweeteners. If you have to eat or drink something that has been sweetened, read your labels carefully.

Other Sources of Toxicity

The Question about Dairy

Dr. Campbell's research and subsequent book, *The China Study* (on dairy and its possible cancer-causing properties) raises a lot of questions about how much dairy (if any) we should have in our diets. Popular opinion would tell you that you need dairy products for the calcium. But there are abundant other rich sources of calcium.

Based on Dr. Campbell's research, I believe that there is reason for caution with milk and milk products, but the danger seems to be dose dependent. Keep dairy consumption lower in your diet to avoid triggering cancer-cell growth. Under 10 grams of protein from dairy a day is probably a safe amount. So if you want yogurt for breakfast, eat it; but that yogurt should be the only dairy you have for the day. Milk with cereal is just a sugar bomb anyway.

Goat cheese and sheep's milk cheese seem to be less carcinogenic (cancer causing) than cow's milk varieties. Try to buy white cheese when possible, so you know that no dye has been used. Beware of "processed cheese food," which is not cheese at all, but purely chemicals.

Obesogens

Obesogens are chemical compounds that cause us to burn fewer calories and predispose weight gain. These substances alter several bodily functions: first, our appetite and feelings of satiety (fullness); second, the regulation of our glucose levels; and third, the regulation of our basal metabolic rate. Research is targeting this phenomenon in order to develop drugs to act as "sort of" anti-obesogens.

Some of the obesogens' chemical compounds are Bisphenol A (BPA), a chemical that is found in plastics (more on that in a minute), and a group of substances called organotins, which include polyvinylchloride plastics, fungicides, pesticides, and wood preservatives.

Two other compounds found in plastic also have been shown to alter the way we store and metabolize fat in our bodies. Those compounds are perfluorooctanoic acid and phthalates.

Plastics

The plastics in pre-packaged food and water bottles contain a number of chemical compounds that can diffuse into the product. The most widely studied thus far is bisphenol A (BPA), which is found in plastic water bottles. In animal testing, BPA has been shown to increase the incidence of some cancers, cause behavioral changes, and decrease immune function. It has been linked to PCOS (polycystic ovarian syndrome), and it is more prevalent in the bloodstream of obese people.

You cannot eliminate every toxic risk in your life, but you can make some changes to limit your exposure. When given a choice, drink from a glass instead of a plastic cup. Try not to allow the plastics that you use to get heated. For example, do not put a plastic container in the microwave. Don't leave water bottles in your car. Opt for a BPA-free bottle. These little things add up when it comes to your health.

PCBs

Polychlorinated biphenyls (PCBs) are an environmental toxin that was used in coolant fluids. Due to their neurologic and endocrine system toxicity, their use has been banned in the United States since 1979. Unfortunately, even though they have been banned for over thirty years, we can still be exposed, most easily from fish in PCB-contaminated waters. In many areas, including the Great Lakes, health advocates recommend that you limit your consumption of fish. Fatty fish caught in industrial areas are the biggest risk.

Fatigue, skin rashes, and coughs are the most common symptoms of PCB exposure. Other effects include disruption of menses in women and possibly infertility. It may increase the risk of certain types of cancer, including estrogen-dependent cancers such as breast cancer and uterine cancer. It also crosses the placenta in a pregnant woman and can affect the fetus with developmental delays.

When it comes to fish, be careful of what parts you eat and know the fish's origin. Never eat the skin, because it concentrates every type of contaminant, not just PCBs. Do not frequently eat fish from a lake in an industrial area. If the fish species is higher on the food chain (that is, it eats lots of other fish), then it is more likely to have higher toxin levels.

In Summary

I am going to beat up on trans fats one more time, because it is that important. Recall that these are chemically altered fats to give foods a longer shelf-life. Another use of trans fats is to prevent oils used for cooking from going rancid. Because trans fats are human-made, your body does not have an inborn mechanism for dealing with them. Their breakdown products basically clog the detoxification system in your body. Trans fats raise your LDL cholesterol and lower your HDL cholesterol. They make your "bad" cholesterol worse and they contribute to heart attacks and stroke.

Read food labels. The two substances you should avoid are trans fats and aspartame. Think about a fast-food meal with a burger, fries, and diet soda. That meal is what you should never eat.

Even when you balance your carbohydrates, proteins, and fats correctly in your diet, it is still important to choose the right source of these macronutrients. When food is in its natural state, it is less likely to contain compounds that are bad for you. Consuming unnecessary calories is not logical for health and weight loss. Don't waste your calories on liquids or foods that are not nutritionally sound. Remember to shop the periphery of the grocery store where fresh foods are kept; if you do so, then making the right choices will be easier.

CHAPTER 7

Overcoming Your Genetics

The age-old question about weight and health is: "Are we genetically programmed to be a certain weight, or is our weight linked to what we eat?" What we have been told is that obesity is the result of an imbalance between the calories we take in and the calories we burn, which results in the storage of energy as fat. But what if weight loss is more complex than that? Obviously, genetic variation accounts for our propensity to either gain weight or lose it.

We all know people we "love to hate"—those people who can eat anything they want and stay skinny. Remember, just because someone is not gaining weight, does not mean he or she is healthy. Our outside appearance does not necessarily reflect the diseases of aging that are developing in our bodies. This chapter will show you the genetic reasons for weight gain and hunger. You will also learn about the role that food allergies play in our overall health. The chapter will also examine the possible future medications to target individual issues with weight loss.

Genetics and Weight

Researchers have been searching for an obesity gene to absolve us of responsibility for the things we eat. Although genetics do play a role, the simple fact is that you still have to play the hand you've been dealt. You can glare at your skinny friend who will cheerfully finish her dessert and then yours, or you can accept that you have to do things differently than she does—and then really do them.

A genetic component to weight gain and loss is most likely going to be polygenic, a term that means that several genes are going to control the physical trait, protein, or hormone imbalance in a given individual. So scientists really aren't looking for just one obesity gene, but probably more like 250, according to one recent report. Research is targeting these genetic variations with drugs. But even if a great pill happens to be made for the problem of being overweight, remember that eating right is not just about weight loss. Weight loss is a just a side effect of Wellness 100. The design of this program is to decrease the damage done to your body internally as you age and maintain a healthy weight.

Nutrition if You Are Expecting a Baby

There is considerable research into metabolic imprinting (or metabolic programming). Basically, this is the theory that a pregnant woman's state of nutrition can have lifelong effects on her baby. This happens at the genetic level in the fetus. What the mother eats or does not eat, and the overall state of her nutrition, could be responsible for turning certain genes on or off for the baby. This process happens as a survival technique for the fetus in utero, but carries through until after birth. The process may affect the child's health throughout life. Animal studies have proven imprinting to have an impact on adulthood obesity, high blood pressure, and insulin resistance leading to diabetes.

I know this may sound scary, which is not my intent. Pregnant women do not have to eat perfectly, but they should consider what they are eating when they are pregnant. (Expectant fathers, be supportive!) Parents should know the long-term effects of their diet on their children. I have been delivering babies for more than ten years, so I see this problem every day. I see mothers who go overboard "eating for two," and mothers who are paranoid about eating anything because they don't want to gain weight. I even see mothers who extinguish their cigarettes on the front porch of my office building before they walk in the door. All of these behaviors could impact a baby for life.

A common-sense approach to nutrition in pregnancy is best. If you think something might be bad for you (such as nicotine, caffeine, additives, preservatives, and so forth), then you probably should not eat it. Strive for fresh foods and lean meats with lots of vegetables, as this program teaches, and don't worry too much about the calories. You need only about 300 more calories per day when you are pregnant. If you are at a comfortable weight and are eating right before you get pregnant, just add a little extra.

How Your Body Interacts with Food

Leptin Levels

Leptin is a protein hormone that helps the body to regulate energy intake through appetite and metabolism. Leptin acts on certain receptors in the brain to inhibit appetite. If you don't have any leptin or there are no receptors for leptin in your brain, your brain never thinks you are full. The result is that you will continue to eat way too much. Leptin levels go up when there is more fatty tissue. So, theoretically, if you have a lot of excess fat tissue, you should not feel hungry. However, obese individuals have much higher levels of leptin than other people. It seems that people can develop leptin resistance, much as people with Type 2 diabetes have insulin resistance. Diets high in fructose and other sugars have been associated with leptin resistance, proving yet again why a high-carbohydrate diet is less satisfying.

There is some early evidence to suggest that melatonin may play a role in leptin levels and/or sensitivity. Melatonin is a hormone made by your body that helps you sleep. Many people take a melatonin supplement at bedtime to help with sleep. Anecdotally, several of my patients have reported feeling less hungry the day after taking melatonin to help with sleep.

Food Responses Among Different People

A new field of nutritional research is emerging called nutritional genomics. Scientists who study this field are focused on deciphering the mechanisms that underlie the interactions between the body and nutrition. They want to know how some people can eat junk all day long and never gain weight. Some interesting information is coming out of this research. For instance, some of the ways our bodies process nutrients are a genetic adaptation that may have helped our ancestors survive. As one example, the HFE gene variant that is associated with a disease called hemochromatosis (in which too much iron builds up in the body) may have given those who possessed this gene a survival advantage in iron-poor regions. We can then see how this adaptation could selectively get passed on. What if the ability to store fat more effectively gave an advantage to people in regions that were prone to famine? Those genes could then be passed down in certain populations, conferring an advantage for survival that is not necessary now.

IgG Food Insensitivities

One of the things that I do as a test with my patients, especially if they hit a plateau or "get stuck" with their weight loss, is a food sensitivity test. Notice this test is a sensitivity test, not an allergy test. An allergy is an IgE reaction in the body that can cause anything from itching, to hives, to anaphylaxis (an allergic reaction that can cause your throat to swell shut). A sensitivity is an IgG reaction by the body to a certain food or spice. With an IgG sensitivity, people may actually crave the foods that they have a reaction to, because they get a little "rush" immediately after eating them. This reaction is the body giving itself a "boost" to neutralize the food quickly. This boost is then followed by a problem an hour or more later, which may last for a day. Or, if the insensitivity involves a food that is eaten frequently, the problem may lead to chronic complaints. These complaints include headaches, fatigue, nausea, irritable bowel syndrome (IBS), foggy thinking, acid reflux, and many others.

I have used IgG testing to break the plateau in weight loss of several of my patients, but one patient in particular, Beth, comes to mind. Beth carried out the program to an extreme, and she ate the same thing for breakfast and lunch every day. She lost 30 pounds very easily, and then she stopped losing for several weeks. We did an IgG test and found that she had sensitivity to peanuts, which she had been eating daily. Once she eliminated them from her diet, her weight loss resumed, and she was able to make her goal weight. She did not have to eliminate them forever, and she could actually have had them once or twice a week. But Beth likes things to be "black and white," so for her, cutting them out worked well.

Another patient, Christine, used to get sushi frequently for lunch. She was suffering from afternoon fatigue and foggy thinking, as well as bloating. A food sensitivity test revealed that she is very sensitive to rice and cucumber, two of the ingredients in her sushi lunch. She stopped eating these foods several times per week, and her energy levels improved.

Blood Type

There is no good scientific evidence to support cutting out a food group based on your blood type. There is evidence, however, that people with different blood types tend to be more sensitive and react negatively to certain foods. People with Type B blood may have more sensitivity to gluten. Those people with Type O may react to seafood. People with a negative blood type have more food sensitivities all around. This information is the only proven data on blood types and food, and these facts have not been tied directly to weight loss.

Research on Diet Drugs

So now you know where diet research is going and what future drugs may target. But what about existing diet drugs, like phenteramine? This drug is an appetite suppressant. It does not melt off weight or speed up your metabolism. Over time, your body gets used to it, and it loses its efficacy as an appetite suppressant. Long-term studies have proven that it does not help people lose weight and keep it off. The weight always comes back, because the person dieting did not learn good habits. These individuals simply cut their caloric intake and then went right back to their old habits.

Another diet pill on the market blocks the absorption of fat in the intestines. The side effects of this pill are increased gas and "uncontrolled anal oil." This drug does not seem to differentiate between the good fats that are healthy for us and the bad ones. Remember that essential fatty acids are called "essential" because we need them to be healthy. What about fat-soluble vitamins? All of these are blocked by the pill from getting into your system as well.

The hcg diet has received a lot of attention lately as a quick way to lose weight. As of this writing, there is no scientific evidence to support this weight-loss approach. When the diet was studied against a placebo, there was no difference in weight loss, fat distribution, or hunger. The mechanism of weight loss with this diet is the 500 calories that they recommend. I do not recommend starvation as a way to lose weight.

Most diet drugs are not conducive to long-term health. We eventually may see drug therapy targeting specific genetic issues or sensitizing our bodies to leptin. Such therapies would help people to lose weight by correcting the underlying errors in the body. But medicine is not to this point yet. When it comes to losing weight, if it sounds too good to be true, it probably is. Yes, life is not fair, and not everyone's body responds the same to foods. You have to learn what your body will tolerate and what your body needs to lose weight. As previously mentioned, this program will not be absolutely perfect for everyone. It will, however, work for just about everyone. Further, this diet will not cause unhealthy side effects while you are losing weight.

CHAPTER 8
Food Selection and Preparation

By now you have a strong grasp of how many and what types of carbohydrates, proteins, and fats to eat. This chapter is intended to show you how to select the best meats and produce. At the end of this book, in Appendix C, there is a shopping list for you to use at the grocery. You will also find out the best ways to prepare foods in order to retain the most nutrients. There are some common misconceptions about food preparation that may surprise you. For instance, I bet you think that grilling is the best way to cook meat. Read on to find out why that is not the case.

These recommendations are the best practices; but as with everything, moderation is the key. You don't have to follow all of these tips every day, but try to keep them in mind and follow them as much as you can.

The Benefits of Organic Foods

It would take another book to discuss all the reasons why organic is better than nonorganic foods. The purpose of this chapter is just to give you an overview. I will focus on the health benefits, but there are environmental benefits as well. For example, there is an increase in wildlife in organic farms, and the soil becomes healthier when it is used to grow organic foods. Further, animals fed organic food are also more fertile. Whether this information holds true for humans remains to be seen.

Organic foods have been shown to be higher in vitamin C, phosphorus, magnesium, iron, and anitoxidants. Additionally, such foods are lower in nitrites and pesticides.

Organic dairy has a better Omega 6 to Omega 3 ratio than dairy that isn't organic. This benefit decreases inflammation throughout the body and therefore decreases diseases of inflammation, including asthma and atherosclerosis.

It is often difficult to tell which fruits and vegetables in the store are genetically modified. There is no mandatory labeling for modified produce. When you buy certified organic, however, that means that the produce will never be items that were genetically modified. So what's the big deal about genetically modified food? Well, many such modified foods are designed to be resistant to the pesticides and herbicides that farmers use. The weeds have now become resistant as well, and farmers are forced to use older, harsher chemicals to control weeds. As the Blue Öyster Cult so eloquently phrased it, "History shows again and again how nature points out the folly of man."

Organic meats eliminate several hassles for you when you are looking for healthy foods. First, with organic meats, you do not have to worry about what the animals were fed and what pesticides the animals consumed. The composition of nutrients in meat is different, depending on how the animal was raised and fed. Most organically raised animals are 100 percent grass fed. This diet for the animal improves the meat's ratio of Omega 6 to Omega 3. Grass-fed beef has been shown to be higher in conjugated linoleic acid (CLA), which fights cancer. When cows are not given their natural diet and are not raised in a healthy habitat, they have to be given antibiotics. We, in turn, consume these antibiotics when we eat meat.

Organic products are more expensive. It may not be possible for you to buy everything organic. If you have to make choices, I would suggest splurging on the organic meat rather than the produce. You can always wash or peel the produce to make it better for you, but you can't do anything to help the meat. Yes, you will be missing out on some of your vitamins; but you should be taking a multivitamin anyway.

The Benefits of Fresh and Seasonal Food

There are many opinions about seasonal and fresh produce, and why it is better for you. Asian traditions tell you that certain foods are either warming or cooling. Summer produce, such as cucumbers and summer squash, are cooling to the body. They provide extra fluids and antioxidants that help with sun exposure. Warming foods like kale, onions, or broccoli, which mature later and store longer, are more nutrient dense and should be consumed more in the fall and winter.

A more Western view of why seasonal is better is that the nutrients start to deplete immediately after harvest. The shorter the time from the farm to the table, the higher the nutrient content. Flavor may be better, too.

Local vs. Organic

When is local better than organic? This topic is becoming a big debate in "foodie" circles. When is it more nutritious and environmentally friendly to eat a local product than something shipped halfway around the world? How much fuel and other resources went into transporting that apple, lettuce, or onion from 3,000 miles away, whereas your local farmer just drove it into the farmers market from 5 miles down the road? Where is the balancing point in nutrition between the time in transport, to the risk of pesticides in the local (but not organic) product? I don't have an answer for this dilemma. I would say just to use your judgment. If you can buy local and know that it was recently harvested, buy it, wash it well, and consume it quickly. Read your labels and buy produce as locally grown as possible. The produce will taste better and retain more nutrients.

Storing Produce

Yes, fresh is best; and if you can go to your local farmers market every day and pick up what you need for dinner, I'm envious! Most of us can't do this. When you can't get fresh, frozen is a good alternative. The process of flash freezing allows most produce to retain its nutritional value. So if given a choice between canned and frozen, go with frozen.

Some foods store better on your countertop and some better in the refrigerator. If you have purchased unripe foods, ripen them in a cool (not cold) place, and then you may refrigerate them. Always store greens, lettuces, berries, mushrooms, broccoli, cauliflower, and asparagus in the refrigerator. You may store cucumbers, eggplant, garlic, ginger, lemons, limes, oranges, apples, and melons on the countertop. Squash, onions, and potatoes should be stored in a cool, dark place. When storing herbs and asparagus, snip off the ends and store them in a jar of water, like a bouquet of flowers.

Food is too expensive to waste. Be sure to plan ahead so that you are able to store your produce properly and use it before it rots. Meats, of course, should be stored in your refrigerator for a couple of days if you plan to use them. Avoid thawing and refreezing. You will lose the moisture that leaked out, and the meat will be drier and less flavorful. If there is too long a period between the thawing and refreezing, you may also be exposing the meat to harmful bacteria and parasites.

How to Cook Meat

The way we cook our meats influences vitamin retention and also affects the possible risk of cancer. Roasting and broiling provide better vitamin retention than stewing. Smaller pieces of meat in stewing provide more surface area where vitamin loss occurs. The "Catch-22" of this issue is that for every 10-degree rise in temperature with cooking, the meal loses twice as much thiamine (vitamin B1); but concurrently, there is a tenfold increase in the destruction of heat-resistant bacteria. It seems that we have a choice to make between the risk of bacteria and the risk of vitamin depletion. That is why cooking fresh, good-quality meats is so important. In general, I recommend cooking better cuts of meat for a longer period, at a lower heat.

There is evidence both for and against high-heat cooking (such as grilling, broiling, and frying), but I think that the most convincing evidence is against it. The most widely studied method is grilling. We have learned that grilling causes the formation of substances called heterocyclic amines. These compounds are commonly found in barbecued beef, chicken, and pork cooked above 392 degrees. The compounds are produced from a combination of high heat, free amino acids (the building blocks of protein), creatine, and sugar. So what do hetercyclic amines do that's bad? They cause mutations in our DNA, which can lead to cancers such as in the breast, prostate, and colon.

Another type of carcinogen is produced by direct-flame grilling. These substances are called polyocyclic aromatic hydrocarbons. So, although the fat may drip away from a flame-broiled burger, you may be better off using a lower-fat ground beef and cooking it on the stove rather than the grill. The newest studies suggest that the risks of grilled meat are highest from the most highly processed varieties, such as hot dogs, sausage, and bacon. If you choose to grill and eat these meats, at least don't grill them to death. Charring your meats to resemble hockey pucks not only makes them taste terrible, but also increases the carcinogenic load.

Smoked meats are even worse. I would recommend that you cut them out of your diet completely. In Iceland, the number of people with stomach and intestinal cancers is the highest in the world. Researchers have blamed this tragedy on the nation's high consumption of smoked fish. The soot from smoking and roasting foodstuffs (such as meat, fish, and coffee) has been shown to be very carcinogenic.

One last note on the high-heat cooking of meats. Researchers at Mt. Sinai Medical Center have found that foods (including meats and vegetables) cooked at high heats form greater levels of advanced glycation endproducts (AGEs). Remember these substances from earlier chapters? They are the substances that can be formed from excess blood sugar, and they cause a variety of issues in the body, including heart disease. These are substances that contribute to physical manifestations of aging such as wrinkles. You can decrease the formation of these substances by not only lowering the temperature while you cook, but also by adding antioxidants to help negate the effects. Good antioxidant foods to use are garlic, onions, and peppers.

Grilling is a quick and easy way to cook, with very little clean up. Do not write grilling off forever because of these risks. What you should take from this information is that grilling should not be the way you cook every night. Reserve this method of cooking for one or two nights per week, so that you decrease your exposure to these potentially harmful substances. Limit your exposure to harmful substances as much as possible, but don't let the issue control your life. You will never be able to cut out all toxic exposures in your life; the best you can do is pick and choose which ones are acceptable risks to you. Charred hot dogs should be something you are willing to give up, but the occasional grilled steak really just makes life worth living!

How to Cook Vegetables

Many alterations occur to vegetables while cooking. These changes can be in texture, taste, color, and overall appeal. Cooking methods also change the vitamin composition of vegetables. The length of time a vegetable is cooked may also contribute to its health benefits. In general, I prefer that you eat them no matter how they are cooked (unless they are boiled to death and covered in processed cheese food, which is just disgusting). Below you will find tips on the best way to prepare your vegetables.

Raw is best. Vegetables in their natural state retain the most vitamins and nutrients. This fact is the main reason that I recommend a salad a day. In a salad, raw vegetables are good. On your plate for dinner, raw vegetables make you feel like you are dieting and depriving yourself of good food. Because Wellness 100 is meant to be a lifestyle, I don't want you to feel deprived.

When onions and garlic are cooked over long periods of time, they lose their nutritional value. To retain as many nutrients as possible, these ingredients should be added at the end. However, this advice is not always the best recommendation for flavor. Just realize that you are not getting all the antibacterial/antiviral properties from garlic if it is cooked for a long time.

Microwave cooking is fast and easy. A 2005 study from India demonstrated that microwaving vegetables does not appreciably change the vitamin content. It does, however, cause greater moisture loss. I usually reserve microwave cooking for warming up leftovers, simply because I don't like how food tastes when cooked in a microwave.

Oils for Cooking

Olive oil is heat stable, which is why it is wonderful for cooking. Heat stable means that it does not change its chemical formula when heated. Never cook with corn oil, poppyseed oil, safflower oil, sesame oil, sunflower oil, or walnut oil. These oils are not heat stable; high heat damages these oils, which in turn damages your body.

Never store a pretty olive oil bottle in a window or above/near your stove. Prolonged exposure to heat and light will damage even olive oil. Always store olive oil in a cool, dark place.

Cookware

If you are in the market for new cookware, some choices seem to be better than others. For instance, cast iron leaks a little iron into your food when you cook with it. It also lasts forever, heats evenly, and it can go from stovetop to oven safely. Ceramic cookware probably does not add anything to your food and it is relatively nonstick.

The verdict is not totally in on Teflon. According to DuPont, the finished product used in nonstick cookware does not contain the harmful chemicals that have been linked to health concerns among factory workers. Personally, I have not thrown out my Teflon-coated cookware, but I am replacing it as it wears out with stainless steel and aluminum.

It Is Up to You to Choose

Learn to make the best choices that your time and budget will allow for your food selection and preparation. No one is perfect all of the time; but when given a choice, remember the guidelines reviewed previously. Careful planning and preparation both helps to eliminate waste of quality foods and ensures that the foods you are feeding yourself and your family are the most nutritious that they can be.

CHAPTER 9

Getting Started with Your Pantry

Stock your pantry and your refrigerator to help you succeed with Wellness 100. You will find that with your healthy eating habits, you are shopping mainly in the meat, produce, and dairy sections of the grocery store. All those aisles in the middle are mainly processed food, which you are avoiding. There are exceptions—some canned items, frozen vegetables, and condiments that you will routinely use—but for the most part, you can shop for and eat fresh food items. Eating healthy will actually save you money, and the end of this section will detail why. First in this chapter you will find a checklist of items to have in your pantry. Then the chapter will provide some detail about the most important items on the checklist. Finally in this chapter, you will read about why eating in a healthy way will save you money.

Items for Your Pantry and Refrigerator

Vegetables

- Buy seasonal, fresh, and local vegetables when they are available.
- Try a mixture of lettuces, such as romaine, spinach, kale, radicchio, leaf, and bib. Variety in your salads adds flavor and keeps your salads interesting, both in taste and visually. You can buy greens already washed and ready to eat, or whole heads. Use your salad spinner to wash and dry several days' worth of salad greens at one time.
- Onions, celery, and carrots—this classic combination of aromatic vegetables is the flavor backbone for many a dish. Buy organic carrots so you can give them a quick wash, and so that you don't have to peel them for soups and cooked dishes. Skip the baby carrots—they are simply large carrots peeled and shaped by machines.
- Avocados
- Tomatoes
- Cauliflower
- Broccoli
- Red and green bell peppers
- Garlic
- Fresh Italian parsley and fresh cilantro—these are two inexpensive herbs used in many recipes. You will be buying them as a bunch. You can cut off about one inch of the stem ends of the bunch. Then place the bunch in water in a tall glass or jar (to help support the herbs). Keep in a cool place on the counter or in the refrigerator.

- Fresh ginger
- Other fresh herbs as indicated in recipes
- Various vegetables according to your meal planning, such as eggplant, zucchini, asparagus, green beans, seasonal squash, and greens

Fruit

- Always have apples and pears on hand. Store apples away from everything else—they cause other produce to ripen faster.
- Buy seasonal fruits that have a low glycemic index, such as blueberries, strawberries, cherries, peaches, and plums.
- Oranges
- One or two lemons and limes
- Only occasionally buy fruit with a higher glycemic index, such as bananas, watermelon, cantaloupe, and dates.

Meat

- Organic meat is always best. If you are going to splurge and buy organic for one group of food, do it for meat.
- Chicken, either whole or breast. Whole, organic chicken is often cheaper than organic pieces.
- Ground turkey and beef—95 percent lean or better
- Fish—buy it fresh and cook it that day or the next
- Lean cuts of beef and meat (see list on page 38)
- Beef for soup and stew (such as sirloin, boneless beef ribs, and beef shank)
- Canadian bacon
- Nitrate/nitrite-free sausage and bacon

Eggs, Cheese, and Dairy

- Eggs
- Hummus (Hummus is not a cheese or dairy product, but it's often found in the dairy section of the supermarket.)
- Sour cream
- Cottage cheese
- Yogurt, Greek (or whole-milk yogurt)
- Heavy cream
- Butter (not margarine)
- Shredded Parmesan (not canned; grated)
- Cream cheese—3 ounce or spreadable

- Feta cheese
- String cheese
- Other high-quality cheese to your liking, such as Asiago or blue cheese, to use in small amounts

Oils, Vinegar, Salad Dressing, Spices, and Condiments
- Extra virgin olive oil
- Vinegar—for salads; stock a variety of balsamic, red wine, white wine, sherry, rice wine, cider, or infused flavored (fig or pear)
- Salad dressings: This book offers you several dressing recipes, starting on page 99. The book also suggests a few commercially prepared salad dressings that have no sugar (or only trace sugar), and other quality ingredients: Annie's Goddess Dressing, Newman's Own—Family Recipe Italian, and Naturally Fresh Ginger Dressing.
- Toasted sesame oil
- Soy sauce
- Dijon-style mustard
- Cumin
- Chili powder
- Whole black pepper and a pepper grinder
- Kosher salt
- Bay leaves
- Dried thyme
- Dried oregano
- Paprika
- Cayenne
- Garlic powder
- Sweet curry powder
- Garam masala
- Other spices as indicated in recipes
- Here's a secret about spices. They are sold, like most food products, in differing qualities and at corresponding price levels. Two mail-order spice companies that offer high-quality spices and herbs in a variety of package sizes are Penzeys (www .penzeys.com) and The Spice House (www.thespicehouse.com). Whatever spices you buy, purchase in quantities that you'll use within a year. Store them in a cool, dry, dark place. When they are no longer aromatic, or seem bitter, discard them.
- You can substitute dried herbs for fresh herbs. Fresh herbs provide a bright flavor and are readily available in most supermarkets today. However, if you choose to substitute dried herbs for fresh, use about 1 teaspoon for every 1 tablespoon of fresh herbs.

Canned and Pickled Supplies

- Chicken, beef, and vegetable broth: Buy preferably organic, low sodium. The recipes here use mainly chicken and vegetable broth.
- Canned tuna
- A variety of canned beans: cannellini, northern, black, and kidney
- Organic diced tomatoes, whole tomatoes, tomato sauce, or pureed tomatoes, preferably in BPA-free cans
- Canned artichokes, whole or quartered
- Chipotle peppers in adobo (small cans)
- Pickles to your liking. If you think you want potato chips, have a pickle instead!
- Olives: green and black Kalamata olives (or tree-ripened black olives)
- Pickled okra, pepperoncini, and so forth to your liking, for use in salads and as snacks
- No-sugar-added peanut butter

Bread, Grains, Sugar, and Starches

- You will notice the absence of flour and sugar on this list. Keep it in small quantities, but you won't have to buy it very often.
- Honey, agave, or stevia as sweeteners
- Panko bread crumbs
- Pasta for use in small quantities (if you desire). Consider couscous (it's easier to portion than other pasta).
- Brown rice and polenta (grits) to use occasionally
- Quinoa (pronounced "keen-wah")
- Dried lentils, green. Red are usually used to make Dal, an Indian dish; green are used in soups and as a side dish.
- Ezekiel bread or 100 percent whole wheat bread
- Whole wheat wraps or sandwich thins
- Corn tortillas—Look for tortillas that have fewer than 15 grams of carbs per tortilla.
- Whole wheat melba toast
- Wasa rye crispbread
- Steel-cut oats or rolled oats

Nuts

- Raw almonds
- Roasted, flavored almonds, such as wasabi (or salt and vinegar)
- Walnuts
- Pine nuts
- Sunflower seeds

- Pistachios
- Cashews

Important Items on the Previous List

Olive Oil

Not only does olive oil make everything taste wonderful, it is great for you. Olive oil is a complex compound made of Omega 3, 6, and 9 fatty acids, vitamins, and several other antioxidant compounds. It is about 85 to 90 percent Omega 9 fatty acid, which is neutral to your body, and 10 percent Omega 6 and 3, which are essential fatty acids. The antioxidants found in the form of flavonoid polyphenols have been shown to lower cholesterol, lower blood pressure, and lower your overall risk of heart disease. Have you heard about the farmers on Crete who consume up to one-half cup per day? They have a low risk of heart disease, despite consuming something that is essentially all fat. Olive oil is also high in vitamins E and K.

Olive oil is good for the stomach. It has been proven to treat ulcers and gastritis. It also stimulates the pancreas and can lower gallstone formation.

The cholesterol formed when consuming large quantities of olive oil is better for you, because it is less likely to become oxidized in your bloodstream. It is now known that oxidized LDL is more damaging to the body's system, leading to more plaque on the arteries.

Olive oil is undamaged by heat during cooking. There are hundreds to choose from, so you can choose the flavor you like best. Always buy extra virgin olive oil. This is from the first cold press. This is olive oil in its most natural state, and it will have retained the best flavor, as well as having the most antioxidants and vitamins.

Nuts

In general, nuts are almost the perfect snack. They are a fantastic mix of carbohydrates, fats, and proteins. They are portable, so you can keep them with you. No crumbs, no sticky mess. If you get really desperate on the go, you can even find them at convenience stores. Keep a variety on hand at home, in your purse or bag, and at work, and you will never be caught snacking on food that you shouldn't! Be careful not to overdo it with nuts. Too much of a good thing is still too much. Try counting out the correct amount and packaging them at home in little Ziploc bags.

Water

Water is not on the pantry list because I assume you have a good supply of drinking water at home. If, however, you do not have good tasting and safe water at home, you should buy it. You should drink the equivalent of half of your body weight in ounces of water per day. If you weigh 160 pounds, you should have 80 ounces of water per day. If you exercise or drink alcohol, you should have more than that.

Be sure to get a BPA-free water bottle and reuse it. In a perfect world, you should keep your water in glass containers instead of plastic. Try filtering water at home, and then storing it in a glass pitcher or jug.

Drinking a large glass of water just before a meal will occupy space in your stomach and make you feel fuller, faster. Also, pause frequently to drink while you are eating. This technique will likely slow down your meal again, helping build the feeling of satiety.

Vitamins

Theoretically, if you are eating well, you shouldn't need vitamins, right? Wrong! Unfortunately, even if you eat absolutely perfectly, you still cannot get all of the vitamins, minerals, and antioxidants your body needs. Modern farming practices have depleted our soil. I am not bashing farmers. For the most part, they don't have much of a choice on how they farm. Again, my father is a farmer, so I really do understand the reality of modern farming. The need to produce more bushels per acre has led to stripping the soil of a lot of nutrients. There is a big movement now toward smaller farms, growing organic produce, and trying to heal the damage that has been done. The reality, however, is that we may not be able to feed the world with that type of farming. Only time will tell.

You should try to buy organic when you can. Organic produce usually has more vitamin content and better mineral content than its nonorganic counterparts. See Chapter 8, which is on food selection and preparation, for more information on organic produce.

I recommend that all my patients take a good multivitamin. Be sure that it is pharmaceutical grade. Vitamins and supplements are not regulated by the FDA; but if you buy pharmaceutical grade, then probably that product is safe and contains what the label says it does.

Spices

Herbs and spices are important for two reasons. First, food that is good for you can also taste good. One of the goals of this book is to teach you that eating healthful is enjoyable. Second, most herbs and spices have a health benefit to them. Eight spices that you will find useful include the following.

1. Black pepper
- Prevents advanced glycation endproducts (AGEs), which are associated with aging and diabetes mellitus (DM). AGEs are the substances that can be formed from excess blood sugar. These substances cause a variety of issues in the body, from heart disease to wrinkles.
- May be a diuretic
- May aid in digestion
- Mild antioxidant

2. Cinnamon
- Prevents advanced glycation endproducts associated with aging and DM
- May lower blood pressure

3. Cloves
- A natural food preservative
- Antibacterial
- Sugar and or increased insulin sensitivity
- May lower LDL cholesterol

4. Cumin
- Prevents advanced glycation endproducts associated with aging and DM
- Aids in digestion
- Antiseptic properties, may help the common cold

5. Curcumin (found in Curry)
- Inhibits angiogenesis (which is necessary for adipose—fat—tissue); thereby facilitates lower body fat and body weight
- India has the lowest rate of Alzheimer's in the world, so it may be that curcumin protects against Alzheimer's.
- Powerful antioxidant
- Anti-inflammatory
- Stimulates flow of bile, and aids in the digestion of fat

6. Garlic
- Antibacterial, antifungal
- Lowers blood sugar
- Lowers blood pressure
- Lowers cholesterol

7. Ginger
- Helps with nausea
- Prevents advanced glycation endproducts associated with aging and DM
- Decreases inflammation, and is good for arthritis
- Is an antioxidant, and therefore may lower cancer risk
- Decreases the glycemic index of sugary foods
- Adding to beans will decrease gassy side effects
- May help with migraines

8. Red Pepper—Capsaicin
- Increases body temperature or heart rate and may increase metabolism
- Decreases lipid oxidation
- May aid in digestion
- Antiseptic properties
- Makes mucus thinner, so may help with lung disorders

Is Eating Healthy More Expensive?

Does it cost more to eat a healthful diet? Why do organic foods cost more, and are they really worth it? To answer these questions, we need to examine the term "cost" from several perspectives. For example, one thing to consider is the actual dollar amount and effect on your grocery bill. Another important factor is the long-term cost of healthcare from not eating in a healthful manner. Finally, there is an overall cost to our environment.

In terms of weekly food costs, let's apply the guidelines of the Wellness 100 program and compare. Organic produce and meats do cost more per pound. When you compare only the price of, for example, an organic avocado, next to the nonorganic one at the store, you may be hesitant to buy the more expensive produce. Remember, however, with Wellness 100 you are learning to cook at home and eliminate waste. With the cheaper avocado, you may be tempted to eat the entire avocado or throw away the unused portion. But after reading this book, you may want to invest in the better avocado (and perhaps an avocado saver for about $5.00) and use the entire fruit in more than one meal. With this program, you should be able eat out less often. You can plan your meals and stock your pantry to be able to use what you have on hand and what is seasonal. We believe that you will likely consume less food, and that you will use your leftovers well. All of these measures will help to decrease your overall food costs.

Portion control, or consuming less food, really affects your budget when it comes to buying meats. A serving of meat should be 4–6 ounces (prior to cooking) and not 8–12 ounces. By cutting back on the amount you are eating, you can reapportion your money and be healthier at the same time. You can still buy larger cuts of meat (a tactic that saves on packaging and is therefore environmentally friendly), and you can eat the leftovers for breakfast or lunch the next day.

You will see a big savings when you eat at home more often and take lunch to work. Pause for a moment to total how much you spend in a week eating out. (Be sure to include beverages and vending snacks.) Apply that number to buying quality produce and meats, and you are likely to experience an actual reduction in food costs.

Eating foods that fill you up and provide energy until your next meal is a strategy that will cause you to snack less. As the following list illustrates, eliminating foods that not only are expensive but also are empty of nutritional value provides savings to be spent on healthier options. Avoid buying junk food (high sugar, low nutritional value), even if it is organic. Unprocessed, real food is the core of Wellness 100.

- Diet soda, especially in those cute small cans, is much more expensive than herbal tea.
- There are about 12 oranges in a 3-pound bag. This is a much better buy than one candy bar.
- A package of cookies can be replaced with fresh fruit, naturally sweet sugar snap peas, or other fresh produce to be incorporated into a meal.

- A bag of chips can be replaced with pickles, hummus, feta cheese (made into a dip for veggies), or raw vegetables.
- It is less expensive to eat an egg than a bowl of name-brand cereal.

Organic produce is more readily available than it used to be, because demand for it today is higher. The difference in price between organic produce and conventional produce is less dramatic today, too, than it was in the past. This price gap will be further reduced as organic farming gains even more in popularity. You may wonder why organic produce costs more. The reason is not because the yields are much smaller from organic farms. Rather, it is higher labor costs associated with organic produce that cause the most difference. Here are two tips that will help you to save money:

1. Buy organic produce that is in season.

2. Buy locally grown.

You will observe that more supermarkets today provide produce that is locally grown or regionally grown. Thus, these two tips help to close the price gap between organic and conventional produce.

The next "cost" associated with your food purchases is the impact to your health. You learned earlier that eating fresh meat and produce (rather than processed food) has big health advantages. Choosing organic produce over nonorganic produce adds another level of benefits. Organic produce has more vitamins, minerals, and antioxidants than nonorganic. These substances are necessary to your overall state of health and your ability to repair the damage that comes from aging and environmental insults. Using organic produce to promote health may decrease your risk of cancer.

Consuming meat, poultry, and dairy without hormones or antibiotics also decreases your risk of major health issues. The higher levels of Omega-3s in organic meats reduce the risk of heart disease. It may be difficult to think of these "savings" when you are filling your grocery cart; but by making the best choices now, you will likely be protecting your body from damage that will lead to more cost in the long run in the form of medical expenses (and suffering).

Finally, let's look at the cost to the environment from conventional farming. (This is a tough subject for me to write about, because as I have said elsewhere in this book, my father is a conventional farmer.) With conventional farming, we are putting a lot of pesticides and herbicides into the environment and into the water supply. Organic farmers have developed new ways (or in some cases, they have resurrected old but savvy methods) to continue to have good yields without using chemicals. One of these techniques is crop rotation to prevent mineral depletion in the soil. Another strategy is to make insectaries (beds of plants at the periphery of the fields); these insectaries serve as habitats for predatory insects.

The recipes in the next section all support the cost-saving tactics of buying seasonal produce, reducing portions, eating at home, and reducing waste. A great resource that you can look up on the internet is an organization called the Environmental Working Group (EWG). They list what foods to buy organic, such as apples and celery. Whether you choose to buy and eat organic produce and meat over conventional products is a personal choice that I hope you will evaluate. Wellness 100 is about making the best choices when it comes to your daily intake of food. Compare, do the math, and decide what is best for you and your family.

Let's Eat! The Recipes

A Message to You from a Passionate Eater

This book, *Wellness 100: 100 Carbs/100 Recipes*, represents a full-circle journey for me. For years I contemplated writing a cookbook to share my passion for cooking and eating, but to what end? What could I offer to friends and family that they could not find on the internet? I considered that I might write about entertaining, such as how to produce glorious meals, brilliantly planned and balanced, full of gastronomic treats.

At the same time, for the first time in my life, I struggled with weight gain. My joints hurt. I suffered from indigestion, and I had puffy eyes and swollen ankles. Dr. Amber French, speaking to me as my doctor and my friend, told me about a wellness program that she had developed to help patients achieve better health through nutrition. I replied, "That sounds great. So many people need that, but I don't need that." I ignored my weight gain, rising cholesterol, and cellulite. I was too busy living large to think about changing my behavior.

A few months later, I went up another size. (So I was living even larger!) I decided that I would not buy bigger clothes again. I looked in the mirror and declared, "I'm nearly fifty years old, and I look it and feel it." In that moment, I knew what I had to do. I called Amber.

I adopted Wellness 100, and so did my husband. Now I eat the right carbs. I buy better meat. I do not drink diet soda. I eat eggs instead of cereal, and I eat a salad a day. I lost eighteen pounds in six months, and my husband lost forty-two pounds. My body is leaner, and my bad cholesterol is lower. Here's the best part: I look better, and I feel better. Even at this point I continue to lose weight, but at a slower pace. I am nearing my set point (my goal weight).

I live to eat, rather than eat to live. Good food has always been important to me. From my viewpoint, that is why Wellness 100 works. First and foremost, Wellness 100 is about eating real food and feeling satisfied after every meal. Eating properly should be nourishing and flavorful; you can have it both ways! That is what I hope to teach you in the following chapters full of appetizing recipes.

These recipes count everything for you. So if you are not used to counting carbohydrates, protein, and calories, begin with the 100 recipes in this book. Soon you won't have to count, because you will know what to eat and how much to eat.

If you are intimidated by the idea of cooking three meals a day, you will find that you won't spend as much time in the kitchen as you feared. These recipes are respectful of your time. Initially, you may need to invest in a few tools. At the grocery store, you will want to start reading labels to know what you are buying and eating. But the payoff comes quickly.

You don't need help indulging; and that's why you won't find recipes here that suggest you can eat dessert every night, as long as you substitute something for something else. If you want to have dessert once in a while, you can choose what's best for you. My goal is to help you stay on course and achieve your goals.

Thank you for choosing the Wellness 100 program. May this program and the recipes in this section become your path to adopting a lifelong habit of eating healthful, flavorful food.

Kari Morris

Cook with Confidence

Tips for Cooking with Wellness 100

- Read the entire recipe before you begin, so that you don't miss important steps or ingredients.

- Assemble and prepare all of the ingredients as directed in the recipe (chop, slice, mince, and so forth) before you begin cooking.

- You can make minor adjustments to heat settings and cooking times as needed. These recipes were developed on a gas stove with a convection oven. Convection ovens generally cook food in less time than a standard oven.

- Make these recipes your own! Have a pen or pencil ready, and modify quantities of seasonings, spices, and herbs to fit your tastes.

CHAPTER 10

Breakfast

Good morning! Most likely you last ate about 12 hours ago, and you need fuel to start the day. You can think of breakfast as "breaking a fast." In the first section, you read that for weight loss and overall wellness, you must eat breakfast, and that you must eat protein and carbohydrates for breakfast.

Include at least 9–10 grams of protein in your breakfast. If you skimp on protein in the morning, you are likely to be hungry before lunch. If you did not get the protein that is required at breakfast, then you would have to boost your protein at lunch or dinner. You have to reach a minimum for the day of 70 grams. It is better to have 9 to 10 grams of protein at breakfast, so that you do not have to load up at lunch or dinner on larger portions of meat and extra calories.

Eggs are the perfect quick breakfast food. It takes no more time to cook an egg, eat it, and rinse out the pan than it does to put on makeup or wait in a fast-food drive-through lane in the morning. You can still eat yogurt and fruit, as long as you avoid sugary yogurts. Instead, buy yogurt of whole milk or Greek yogurt. A bowl of cereal is not part of a balanced breakfast, but breakfast can include oats that are whole grain (such as steel-cut oatmeal).

If you must have a "breakfast to go," then you can make an egg sandwich. Or you can take a piece of fruit and a hard-boiled egg or two. Or you can make a smoothie. The recipes in this chapter give you many options to "eat in" or "take with."

At breakfast, you should consume 20 to 30 percent of your total calories for the day. According to the calorie chart on page 5, a 45-year-old, 5'5" tall woman should eat 250 to 375 calories at breakfast—but only 120 of these calories should be from carbohydrates (30 grams × 4 calories per gram).

Easy Eggs for Breakfast

You can cook eggs a number of ways to suit your lifestyle and your tastes. Table 10.1 provides instructions for quick cooking methods, easy to accomplish on busy mornings.

Because you need carbohydrates as well as protein, you can eat eggs with a piece of whole wheat bread (or corn tortilla) and a piece of fruit. Boost your protein intake by adding meat, such as a small portion of cooked meat from your meal the previous night. (Even though you are reducing your meat portions at dinner, prepare enough to have for breakfast or lunch the next day.) Limit your intake of traditional breakfast meats, such as bacon and sausage. They are high in saturated fat, and they have nitrites and often sugar.

1 egg = 0 carbs, 6 protein, 80 calories

Table 10.1
Six Quick Ways to Make Eggs

Style	Method	Ideas
Fried Eggs It takes no longer to fry an egg than it does to make toast.	Heat a heavy pan or nonstick pan over medium-low heat. Add 1 teaspoon of olive oil. Add an egg. Cook for one minute, then flip with a spatula, and cook for 1 more minute. Season with salt and pepper.	If you don't like to flip eggs, try this method. After adding the egg to the pan, add about 2 teaspoons of water to the pan and cover. Cook to desired doneness (about 3 minutes for medium).
Scrambled Eggs The key to fluffy scrambled eggs is to use low heat and stir gently. High heat = dry eggs!	Heat 1 teaspoon of olive oil in a small pan over medium-low heat. Crack 1 or 2 eggs into a small bowl, add a teaspoon of water, and beat lightly. Add beaten eggs to the pan, and allow eggs to set slightly. Use a spatula to stir gently.	Some classic additions to scrambled eggs include heavy cream and cream cheese (just a bit), chopped chives or green onions, fresh tarragon, dill, dried marjoram, or cayenne and nutmeg.

Style	Method	Ideas
Hard-boiled Eggs This is a great "on the go" breakfast choice. One boiled egg and a small smoothie or piece of fruit can get you going. Boiled eggs are portable, long lasting, and are cooked without added fat for a great weight loss option.	Place eggs in a single layer in a large saucepan. Add cold water to cover the eggs. Bring to a boil over medium-high heat, remove from the heat, and cover. Let sit for 15 minutes. Use tongs or a slotted spoon to transfer the hot eggs to a bowl of ice water. After about 10 seconds, you can handle the eggs to gently crack the shells (do not peel). Return eggs to the cold water to cool them completely. Remove the eggs from the water. You can store the cracked, but unpeeled, eggs in the refrigerator for up to a week.	Hard-boiled eggs aren't just for breakfast. You can use them in salads, as a snack, as part of an appetizer plate, or as a garnish for soups.
Stove-top Frittatas Frittatas are an easy one-pot meal.	Cook the meat and vegetables first over medium heat. Then turn the heat to low and add lightly beaten eggs and herbs as desired. Cover. Cook until the eggs are set, about 5 minutes.	Use leftover grilled or roasted vegetables for a quick frittata. Add small amounts of meat to your frittatas for flavor and protein. See the recipes beginning on page 90.
Breakfast Tacos Use corn tortillas instead of flour tortillas.	Fluffy scrambled eggs are not required for breakfast tacos—cook it, fill it, eat it, and away you go!	Try a double-meat taco without eggs for a high-protein breakfast.
Poached Eggs Poached eggs have no added fat, and the yolks are perfect for dipping with whole wheat toast. Eggs can be poached in the microwave. Check the microwave manual for directions specific to your brand. If you have lost the manual, it may be available online.	Use a skillet with straight sides or a sauce pan. Fill the pan with water to a depth of at least 2 inches. It's easier to poach eggs in deeper water. Add 1 tablespoon of white vinegar to the water. Bring the water to a slow simmer. Crack the eggs into a ramekin, then tip the ramekin into the water to deposit the egg gently. The egg will drop to the bottom, then float up as it cooks.	Poached eggs generally take 3 to 4 minutes to cook. Use a slotted spoon to remove the eggs from the water and to drain the egg before serving.

Fast Fried Egg and Meat Breakfast

This nutritional breakfast is fast, because you don't have to cook the Canadian bacon–you are just warming it. This combination of protein and carbohydrates will keep you going until lunch.

1 serving

1	egg
1	teaspoon extra virgin olive oil
1	piece Ezekiel bread (or whole wheat bread)
2	slices Canadian bacon (or other meat options as given below)
1	medium orange (or an appropriate portion of another fruit)

Heat a small (8-inch) skillet, over medium-low heat. Drop bread into the toaster. Add olive oil to the pan. Add Canadian bacon to the pan, just to warm it (this step takes less than one minute) and remove the bacon from the pan. Crack one egg into a pan. Fry to your liking. Toast is up–now that's fast!

Other meat options include thinly sliced leftover steak or pork. Or you could have two homemade breakfast sausage patties (see page 85).

Save calories and don't butter your toast. The reason is because 1 teaspoon of butter contains 33 calories but offers you no appreciable protein or carbs.

Nutrition Analysis: 31 carbs, 22 protein, 332 calories

"To-Go" Sandwich with Hummus

Use two pieces of whole wheat bread. Spread the bread with ½ tablespoon of hummus. Add a cooked egg and a piece of heated Canadian bacon, and out you go (no fruit).

Nutrition Analysis: 27 carbs, 26 protein, 356 calories

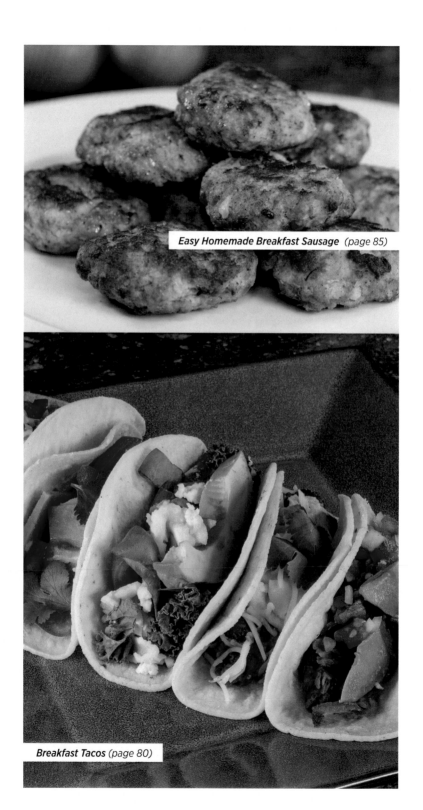

Easy Homemade Breakfast Sausage (page 85)

Breakfast Tacos (page 80)

Breakfast Tacos

Breakfast tacos provide a hearty, flavorful breakfast in no time. Be careful not to overload your breakfast tacos, however, because breakfast is one meal where it is very important to watch calories, especially if weight loss is your goal. You need not eat eggs every day, and a "double-meat," eggless breakfast taco is a great way to get your protein using warmed beef, chicken, or pork from last night's dinner.

Per person

1   **egg, beaten**
     Vegetables, fresh or cooked
2   **corn tortillas (or 1 small, whole wheat wrap), warmed**
1   **ounce meat. You can use homemade breakfast sausage (page 85), leftover meat (cut into strips), or chili. Another option is to use ¼ of an avocado.***

Heat a small (8-inch) frying pan, over medium-low heat. Add meat to cook or reheat. Add the egg and stir to scramble. Place the egg and meat mixture into warm tortilla(s). Top with salsa and fresh vegetables. Choose from among these optional fillings and garnishes:

- sliced or chopped tomato
- fresh spinach leaves
- green or red bell peppers, thinly sliced
- fresh onion, thinly sliced

- jalapenos, fresh or pickled
- salsa
- cilantro
- crumbled feta (1 tablespoon)

*You can see from Table 10.2, "Nutritional Analysis for Breakfast Tacos," that breakfast tacos in many combinations fall within the limits of a healthy breakfast. To limit your calories for weight-loss purposes, you may need to choose either meat or avocado, but not both in the morning.

Table 10.2
Nutrition Analysis for Breakfast Tacos

Ingredients	Carbs	Protein	Calories
scrambled egg	0	6	80
meat (1 ounce)	0	8	53
nitrate-free bacon, 2 slices, cooked	0	6	92
¼ avocado	4	1	80
fresh veggies	2	0	8
feta cheese	0	1	25
corn tortilla (2)	22	2	104
whole wheat wrap (1)	16	2	120
olive oil (1 teaspoon)	0	0	40
Combination Tacos	**Total Carbs**	**Total Protein**	**Total Calories**
1 egg, meat, avocado, veggies, 2 corn tortillas	28	17	365
1 egg, meat, veggies, cheese, 2 tortillas (no avocado)	24	17	310
1 egg, avocado, 2 tortillas (no meat, no cheese)	26	9	304
1 egg, avocado, veggies, cheese, 2 tortillas	28	10	337
no eggs, double meat, veggies, cheese, 2 tortillas	24	17	243

Scrambled Egg with Ricotta, Avocado, and Tomato

1 serving

1	teaspoon extra virgin olive oil
1	egg
2	tablespoons whole-milk ricotta
¼	cup chopped tomato (or cherry tomatoes cut in half)
¼	avocado, chopped or sliced

Lightly beat the egg and mix in the ricotta cheese. Blend the egg and cheese. Heat olive oil in a small (8-inch) frying pan, over medium-low heat. Cook the tomatoes just to heat them, then reduce some of the liquid. Add the egg and ricotta mixture. Cook to desired doneness. Top with the chopped or sliced avocado.

Optional: Garnish with fresh basil, parsley, or cilantro.

Nutrition Analysis: 7 carbs, 12 protein, 262 calories

Add 23 more carbs to your breakfast with a piece of fruit, and you have 354 calories in your meal.

> **Avocados** are good for the skin. They contain Omega 3 fatty acids that help the skin from drying out. Avocados also may reduce ultraviolet (UV) damage from sun exposure.

Creamy Eggs with Canadian Bacon and Tomato

1 serving

1	teaspoon olive oil
1	egg, beaten
2	teaspoons cream cheese
½	small tomato, coarsely chopped
1	slice Canadian bacon, chopped (or a small portion of cooked steak or pork)
	Salt and freshly ground, black pepper

Mix the cream cheese into the beaten egg. (Lumps of cream cheese will remain, but these lumps will melt during cooking.)

Heat olive oil in an 8-inch frying pan, over medium-low heat. Add the tomato to the pan and cook until most of the liquid has evaporated. Season with salt and pepper. Reduce heat to low. Add the Canadian bacon, egg, cheese, and basil mixture. Stir over low heat to desired doneness.

Nutrition Analysis: 2 carbs, 13 protein, 195 calories

Add whole wheat toast (or fruit) to reach 30 carbs.

Peanut Butter Breakfast Sandwich

No-sugar-added peanut butter and almond butter are acceptable forms of protein in the morning, but these ingredients have their limitations. It takes 2 tablespoons of either to provide about the same amount of protein in 1 egg, but those 2 tablespoons have more than twice the calories of 1 egg (about 190 calories). Fruit and cinnamon create a great morning flavor combination.

1 serving

1	piece Ezekiel or whole wheat bread, toasted
	Ground cinnamon
2	tablespoons no-sugar-added peanut butter (or almond butter)
¼	large apple, thinly sliced (or an equal amount fresh apricot or peach)

Spread the peanut butter over toast. Top with sliced fruit and sprinkle with cinnamon.

Nutrition Analysis: Nutrition Analysis: 29 carbs, 11 protein, 299 calories

Easy Homemade Breakfast Sausage

Why take the time to make your own breakfast sausage? The answer becomes "Why not?" when you consider that it has less saturated fat compared to regular breakfast sausage. It has no nitrites and is cost effective. Because it is easy to make, you can make a batch of sausage and then freeze the patties for busy weekday mornings. Just thaw patties in the refrigerator the night before, reheat, and enjoy on an egg sandwich. Patties are super as a side, or in breakfast tacos, frittatas, or scrambled eggs.

Makes 10 to 15 servings, which is thirty patties.

	Extra virgin olive oil for cooking
1	pound ground pork
1	pound ground turkey
¼	cup minced onion
1	tablespoon rubbed sage
2	teaspoons Kosher salt
1	teaspoon dried thyme, crushed between your fingers
¼	teaspoon cayenne pepper
1	teaspoon crushed red pepper
¼	teaspoon ground allspice

In a small bowl, blend the sage, salt, thyme, cayenne, crushed red pepper, and allspice.

In a large bowl, add the ground pork, ground turkey, and minced onion. Mix well with a large spoon or with your hands. Add the spice mixture to the meat mixture, and work the spice mixture into the meat to blend it well.

In a small frying pan, heat 1 teaspoon of extra virgin olive oil and cook a small portion of the sausage mixture. Taste; if needed, add more seasonings to the uncooked sausage mixture. For instance, add more crushed red pepper or cayenne if you like spicier sausage.

Portion and shape the sausage mixture into 1-ounce patties, about 1 ½ inches in diameter and ½-inch thick.

Heat 1 tablespoon of extra virgin olive oil in a large skillet, over medium heat. Add the sausages in batches, not crowding the pan. Brown on both sides and cook through. Cool the sausage patties and wrap them in portions. Label, date, and freeze. When you need them, thaw them overnight in the refrigerator and reheat them in a frying pan with a little bit of olive oil.

Nutrition Analysis:
2 patties: 1 carb, 10 protein, 129 calories
3 patties: 2 carbs, 16 protein, 193 calories

Cold Ham and Egg Breakfast Sandwich

1 serving

1	hard-boiled egg, peeled and sliced
2	ounces Black Forest Ham (or other deli ham)
	Dijon-style mustard
2	slices whole wheat bread
1	slice fresh tomato

Smear a small amount of Dijon-style mustard on the bread. Top the bread with ham, tomato, and the boiled egg. Season with black pepper.

Nutrition Analysis: 29 carbs, 23 protein, 329 calories

Fruit and Peanut Butter Smoothie

You can still have smoothies for breakfast. Just realize that this yogurt drink accounts for an entire day's worth of dairy. For added protein and long-term energy, add peanut butter or protein powder to the blender. Blend in a blender until smooth.

1 serving

½   cup yogurt (whole milk or Greek)
1   tablespoon no-sugar-added peanut butter or almond butter
     Fruit portioned to equal approximately 22 carbs:
     1   small apple, or
     1   heaping cup blueberries, or
     1   large peach, or
     1½   cups blackberries

Nutrition Analysis:
Greek yogurt: 30 carbs, 13 protein, 333 calories
Plain, whole-milk yogurt: 32 carbs, 8 protein, 258 calories

Greek-style yogurt has been strained to remove the whey, which makes it thicker and smoother. It is higher in protein and lower in carbs than other yogurts.

High-protein Granola

High-protein Granola is lower in carbohydrates and higher in protein than most store-bought granola, because it uses more nuts and seeds than most commercially prepared versions. It also has fewer oats and less sugar.

Makes 4 cups (16 servings)

1 ½	cups old-fashioned rolled oats
1	cup raw almonds, chopped
½	cup sunflower seeds
½	cup walnuts, chopped
½	cup sweetened coconut
¼	cup no-sugar-added peanut butter
2	tablespoons canola oil
½	teaspoon pure vanilla extract
⅛	teaspoon pure almond extract
½	teaspoon ground cinnamon

Preheat the oven to 300°F. Spray a rimmed baking sheet with cooking spray.

Mix the oats, almonds, sunflower seeds, walnuts, and coconut in a large bowl. In a small bowl, mix the peanut butter with the canola oil, vanilla, almond, and cinnamon. Pour the peanut butter mixture over the oat mixture and stir to coat evenly. Spread the mixture on the baking sheet and bake for about 10 minutes. Stir. Cook another 10 minutes or until the nuts are toasted. Be careful not to burn the granola.

Serving size: ¼ cup
Nutrition Analysis: 10 carbs, 5 protein, 176 calories

With yogurt and fruit: Served with ½-cup whole-milk yogurt and an appropriate serving of fruit, your breakfast is 30 carbs, 10 protein, and about 330 calories.

Egg and Black Bean Tostadas

This dish is inspired by huevos motulenos, a Mexican breakfast consisting of refried pinto beans, ham, fried eggs, and peas served on a corn tortilla with ranchero sauce (which does make a nice breakfast, too). Perhaps this dish is a bit involved for a workday morning, but these egg tostadas are worth the effort on your day off. The black beans, spinach, and egg create a satisfying combination.

2 servings

2	eggs
4	corn tortillas
	Fresh spinach leaves
	Fresh salsa (page 114)
½	avocado, chopped or sliced (each plate gets ¼ avocado)
2	tablespoons feta cheese
	Chopped, fresh cilantro or parsley
¼	cup refried black beans, cooked as noted in the following (each plate gets 2 tablespoons of cooked beans)

To make the refried black beans, rinse and drain 1 (14-ounce) can of black beans. Heat 2 tablespoons of olive oil in a small, nonstick frying pan, over medium-low heat. Add the black beans and stir. When the beans are heated, mash them with a rubber spatula until the beans are smooth. Do not overcook the beans, or they will dry out. (If they do become dry, add a bit of water to refresh them.) Remove the beans from the heat. If you like chipotle peppers, you can add a spoonful of the sauce (or more to your liking) from chipotle peppers in adobo to the refried beans. (Adobo means sauce or mixed seasonings.)

In a separate pan, fry the eggs. Warm the corn tortillas.

Stack two tortillas on each of two plates. Top the tortillas with two tablespoons of refried beans and spread the beans to cover the tortillas. Put a small mound of fresh spinach leaves on top of the refried beans. Top the spinach with the fried eggs. Top the eggs with the salsa, avocado, feta, and cilantro or parsley.

Save the leftover beans to add to a sandwich wrap or to a soup as a thickener. Or, you can eat the leftover beans with a fried egg the next day.

Nutrition Analysis: 32 carbs, 12 protein, 308 calories

Stove-top Frittatas

A frittata is nothing more than an unfussy omelet—no folding required! Cook some fillings of your choice, then bind them together with 2 beaten eggs. Frittatas are a good way to use leftover meat and vegetables, a tactic that reduces your preparation and cooking time on busy mornings. Frittatas (like omelets) also make a nice lunch or dinner with a mixed-greens salad with vinaigrette.

I find frittatas are hard to make with only 1 egg, because the egg spreads out too thin in an 8-inch frying pan. If you are making a frittata for one person, use two eggs; and if you are serving two people, three eggs will suffice.

2 servings

2   eggs, beaten, or 3 eggs for two people
¾ to 1 cup coarsely chopped, fresh (or previously
          cooked) vegetables
1 or 2 ounces meat (such as steak or pork)
1   teaspoon extra virgin olive oil
        Salt and freshly ground, black pepper
        Garnish of fresh parsley (or a bit of grated cheese)

You can double this recipe to feed 4 people: use 6 to 8 eggs and a 10-inch skillet.

Heat 1 teaspoon of olive oil in an 8-inch frying pan, over medium heat. (As you can see in the following, you may want to use an oven-proof skillet.)

Frittatas often are started on the stove top and finished in a hot oven or broiler. You can do that, too. Preheat the oven to 425°F before you begin to cook, or turn on the broiler. Use an oven-proof skillet. After you lift the egg in Step 5, place the skillet in the oven to "set" the top of the frittata (about 1 minute under a broiler, or 3–5 minutes in a hot oven).

1. Cook the raw meat. Degrease the pan if necessary. Then add any uncooked vegetables and cook until soft, but not brown.
2. If you're using already-cooked meat, then heat the meat and vegetables in olive oil together.
3. Pour the beaten eggs over the meat and vegetables. Season with salt and freshly ground, black pepper.
4. Turn the heat to low and cover the pan.
5. After the eggs begin to set (in about 2 minutes), lift the edge of the eggs and tilt the pan to allow the uncooked eggs to fill-in underneath. Cover the pan and cook the mixture until the eggs are set (about 5 more minutes).
6. Larger frittatas will require a bit more cooking time. You also would perform another "lift" maneuver to allow the uncooked eggs to fill-in underneath.
7. Garnish the meal with fresh herbs and/or grated cheese, if desired.

Serve the frittatas with an appropriate portion of fruit or toast to reach 30 carbs.

Roasted or Grilled Vegetable Frittata

Use leftover roasted or grilled vegetables from your dinner the night before, such as cauliflower, onions, asparagus, squash, zucchini, mushrooms, peppers, eggplant, or sweet potatoes.

1 serving

¾	cup coarsely chopped, cooked vegetables
1	teaspoon extra virgin olive oil
2	eggs, beaten
	Salt and freshly ground, black pepper
2	teaspoons chopped, fresh basil or parsley (optional)
1	tablespoon grated Parmesan cheese (optional)

Heat 1 teaspoon of olive oil in an 8-inch frying pan, over medium-low heat. Add the vegetables to warm them. Season with salt and freshly ground, black pepper. Beat the 2 eggs. Pour the eggs over the vegetables, then turn the heat to low and cover the pan. After 2 minutes, lift the edges of the frittata to allow the uncooked eggs on top to fill-in underneath. Cover the pan and cook the mixture until it is set.

Sprinkle with optional fresh herbs and Parmesan cheese.

Nutrition Analysis: 6 carbs, 16 protein, 247 calories

Option: You can add 1 ounce of cooked leftover steak or pork. Simply add in the calories, which is approximately 57 calories (for a total of 304 calories).

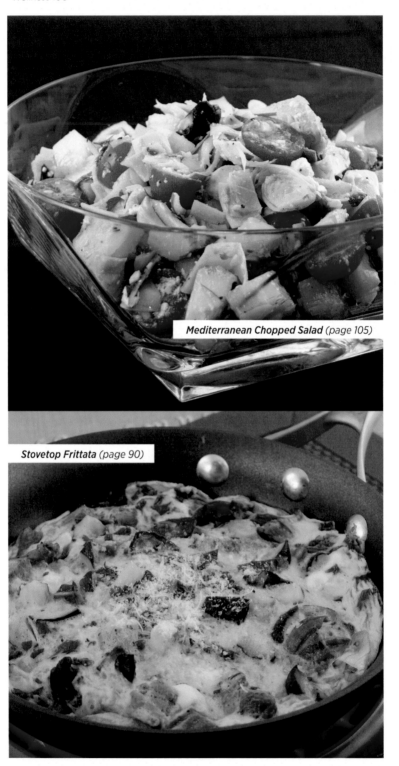

Mediterranean Chopped Salad (page 105)

Stovetop Frittata (page 90)

Spinach and Artichoke Frittata

1 serving

1   teaspoon extra virgin olive oil
2   eggs, beaten
1   tablespoon heavy cream
¼   cup artichoke hearts, coarsely chopped (about 2 hearts from a 14-ounce
         can; the rest you can refrigerate in their liquid in a non-metal container for
         another use)
½   cup (packed) fresh spinach leaves
         Fresh lemon juice

Coarsely chop the artichoke hearts and add a small bit of lemon juice (to stop discoloration when cooking). Heat the olive oil in an 8-inch skillet, over medium-low heat. Add the artichokes and cook for about 1 minute.

Add the cream and spinach leaves to the beaten eggs, and mix thoroughly. Season with salt and freshly ground, black pepper. Pour the egg mixture into the pan with the artichokes, then turn the heat to low and cover the pan. After 2 minutes, lift the edges of the eggs to allow the uncooked egg mixture on top to fill-in underneath. Cover the pan and cook the mixture until set.

Nutrition Analysis: 7 carbs, 13 protein, 249 calories

Ham and Asparagus Frittata

1	teaspoon extra virgin olive oil
2	eggs, beaten
2	ounces ham (or Canadian bacon), coarsely chopped
¾	cup asparagus, trimmed, sliced into 1-inch pieces
2	tablespoons freshly grated Parmesan cheese
	Dash dried tarragon

Add ½ inch of water to an 8-inch frying pan. Bring the water to a simmer over medium-high heat. Add the asparagus and cook the asparagus until it is just tender, about 3 minutes. Remove the asparagus and drain any remaining water from the pan.

Reduce the heat to medium low, and add 1 teaspoon of olive oil to the pan. Add the ham and asparagus, cooking just enough to heat the ham. Mix the cheese and tarragon into the eggs. Season with freshly ground, black pepper. Reduce the heat to low, and pour the egg mixture over the ham and asparagus. Cover the pan. After 2 minutes, lift the edges of the eggs and tilt the pan to allow any uncooked egg mixture on top to fill-in underneath. Cover the pan and cook until set.

Nutrition Analysis: 4 carbs, 29 protein, 270 calories

Eat Protein with Oatmeal

Oatmeal is a good option as a Wellness 100 breakfast food. All oatmeal is not equal, however. You can make an informed choice as to which types of oatmeal to keep in your pantry. It is good to know the role that oatmeal plays in your diet.

A serving of oatmeal typically provides all of your carbs for breakfast, but not enough protein. Plan to add a hard-boiled egg or a portion of meat on the side. As a reminder, if you do not eat enough protein for breakfast, you are likely to be hungry by mid-morning. Another thing that would happen if you did not eat enough protein for breakfast is that you would need to eat more protein later in the day to reach 70 grams. But you do not want to eat more protein later in the day, because doing so equates to a larger portion of meat at one sitting.

Generally speaking, the more refined (or processed) oats are, they quicker they cook. But more refined oats have a higher glycemic index and a lower protein content. Less-refined oats take longer to cook, but they have more soluble fiber, a lower glycemic index, and more protein. Avoid instant oatmeal and never eat the flavored instant oatmeal with added sugar.

Oatmeal Options

Best	Steel-cut oats
Okay	Rolled oats
Avoid	Instant oatmeal
Never	Flavored (sugar-added) instant oatmeal

The downside of steel-cut oats is that they require up to 20 minutes to cook after they have come to a boil. Try cooking a large batch early in the week or on Sunday. You can refrigerate the oatmeal for up to 3 days, and you can reheat single servings.

Read labels carefully. One packet of instant oatmeal contains only 17–19 carbs; but the portion is smaller than a single serving of rolled or steel-cut oats, and it contains no soluble fiber. It's not a good trade-off.

CHAPTER 11

A Salad a Day

An important component of the Wellness 100 program is to eat a salad a day. Fresh salads, made up of mainly raw vegetables, contribute more vitamins and minerals to your diet than cooked vegetables. Because one cup of lettuce contains less than 10 calories, these recipes don't include portions for lettuce and other fresh greens. You can eat what you like, as long as you aren't loading your lettuce with lots of cheese or sweet dressings.

Whether the salad is the meal, or a side dish to a meal, it need not be cumbersome to make. A few fresh ingredients paired with an appropriate dressing give salads a wonderful balance of flavors, textures, and visual appeal. Salads easily lend themselves to seasonality, too, which means you can take advantage of what's fresh now and enjoy tasty and local produce year-round.

Keep a variety of salad greens in your refrigerator to add texture and color to your salads. I always keep romaine, and then I have either spinach or kale. I also have radicchio or some sort of cabbage. I often chop a small portion of all of these greens into my salads. You can also shred or thinly slice Brussels sprouts into a salad. Brussels sprouts are delicious and slightly bitter; you can remove any wilted outer leaves before shredding. Avoid iceberg lettuce, because it is lower in almost all vitamins and minerals, compared to other salad greens.

Perhaps your dinner already includes meat and vegetables. In that case, assembling a side salad is as easy as topping fresh greens with olive oil and vinegar. If you want to get fancier than that, in this chapter you will find recipes for homemade dressings, several side salads that incorporate a variety of vegetables, and salads that make a meal. Here are a few tips for adding "a salad a day" into your meal planning:

Use a salad spinner. Fill the bowl and basket with cold water. Cut your salad greens, or use whole leaves and add to the water to wash well. Lift the basket to drain the greens. Pour out the water, and replace the basket; then attach the spinner top and spin. Now your lettuce is dry and will be crisper, will last longer, and will hold dressing better. Store clean, spun lettuce in a covered container lined with a paper towel, and it will keep for 3 to 5 days for easy access.

Fresh vegetables that add crunch and natural sweetness to a salad include sugar snap peas, jicama, carrots, fennel bulb, and red, green, or yellow peppers.

- Wash and cut extra fresh vegetables for lunch salads and snacks during the week. Celery and carrots keep well in ice cold water. Other veggies should be washed and dried, then sliced and stored in a container with a lid. Line the container with a paper towel to absorb any extra moisture.

- Make to-go lunch salads the night before, but do not dress the salad. If you are leaving for work, pack a dressing and crunchy toppings (such as nuts or sunflower seeds) separately to add just before eating.
- Use leftover baked, roasted, or grilled meat in your lunch salads. Even though you are reducing your meat portions at dinner, prepare enough to have for lunch the next day.
- Boiled eggs, canned tuna, deli ham or turkey, nuts, and beans also add protein to your salads.

Remember to eat your side salad as a first course if you want to calm a fierce appetite. Doing so will help you to control portions.

Salad Dressings

The most simple and one of the most satisfying salad dressings is a mixture of high-quality, extra virgin olive oil and balsamic vinegar. Toss your salad first with olive oil and a dash of salt and pepper. Then sprinkle on vinegar to taste. For variety, this book offers you several dressing recipes. The recipes also use some commercially prepared salad dressings that have no sugar (or only trace sugar) and other quality ingredients. Three of our favorites are Annie's Goddess Dressing, Newman's Own—Family Recipe Italian, and Naturally Fresh Ginger Dressing.

Use lighter, more delicate dressings with more delicate greens, and employ zestier dressings with bolder or peppery greens.

This book's nutrition analysis allows a generous 2 tablespoons of salad dressing per serving. The book's dressings include very small amounts of carbohydrates (in the form of vinegar, citrus juice, or honey). Because you should eat 2 tablespoons of olive oil a day, you can't overindulge these homemade salad dressings. Remember—when you adhere to the requirements for protein and carbs, you can let the good fat (like olive oil) fall into place. So no worries!

Versatile Vinaigrettes

Many store-bought dressings are full of corn syrup, sugar, or preservatives. These dressings are in your past! Classic vinaigrette is easy to whip together, and the options are endless. Here are several ideas for versatile vinaigrettes.

Classic Vinaigrette

Serving size: 2 tablespoons

- ¼   cup red-wine vinegar (or white-wine vinegar)
- ½   teaspoon Dijon-style mustard
- ¼   teaspoon salt
- ¼   teaspoon freshly ground, black pepper
- ½   cup extra virgin olive oil

In a medium bowl, whisk the first four ingredients to blend: vinegar, mustard, salt, and pepper. Continue whisking and add the olive oil in a slow, steady stream. Whisk until the mixture is blended. Cover the bowl and refrigerate it. If the dressing separates, whisk it again before using. Most vinaigrettes keep up to a week in the refrigerator, so make a double batch to have it on hand for your salads.

Nutrition Analysis: 0 carbs, 0 protein, 163 calories

Variations
Balsamic Vinaigrette
Prepare as directed, but substitute balsamic vinegar for the red-wine vinegar.
Shallot Vinaigrette
Prepare as directed, but add 2 tablespoons of minced shallots before whisking in the olive oil.
Lemon Vinaigrette
Prepare as directed, but substitute fresh lemon juice for the red-wine vinegar. If you like capers, add 1 tablespoon of rinsed, chopped capers.
Fresh Herb Vinaigrette
Prepare as directed, using white-wine vinegar instead of the red-wine vinegar. Stir in 1 tablespoon of fresh chives and 1 teaspoon of chopped, fresh tarragon, or your favorite herb.

Greek-style Dressing

If you find the garlic taste too strong in this recipe, add more lemon juice and olive oil; the next time you make it, you can modify the recipe. I like a bold garlic presence with certain salads, especially Greek salads, and so I use a whole clove.

Serving size: 2 tablespoons

¼	cup fresh lemon juice
1	teaspoon Dijon-style mustard
1	teaspoon dried oregano
1	small clove garlic, pressed or minced
¼	teaspoon salt
¼	teaspoon freshly ground, black pepper
⅓	cup extra virgin olive oil
2	tablespoons chopped, fresh parsley

Garlic is rich in antioxidants. It is said to be a natural remedy to the common cold, perhaps because it enhances our immune system.

When you are using fresh lemon juice in a dressing, grate some of the lemon peel before juicing. You can add the grated peel to the dressing (or directly to the salad) for a bright, lemony taste.

In a medium bowl, whisk together the lemon juice, mustard, oregano, garlic, salt, and pepper. Continue whisking and add extra virgin olive oil in a slow, steady stream until the mixture is well blended. Stir in the fresh parsley. Cover the bowl, and refrigerate it. The flavor of garlic may intensify over time, so it is best to use this dressing within a day or two.

Nutrition Analysis: 1 carb, 0 protein, 110 calories

Sesame Dressing

Serving size: 2 tablespoons

½   cup balsamic vinegar
1   clove garlic, pressed or minced
1   tablespoon honey
2   tablespoons lemon juice
     Salt and freshly ground, black pepper
¾   cup extra virgin olive oil
¼   cup toasted sesame oil

In a medium bowl, whisk together the vinegar, garlic, honey, lemon juice, salt, and pepper. Continue whisking; add olive oil and then sesame oil in a steady stream. Whisk until the mixture is well blended.

Nutrition Analysis: 4 carbs, 0 protein, 154 calories

This recipe is fairly high in carbs, compared to other dressings. Why? Because balsamic vinegar is made either by concentrating late-harvest grape juice (the traditional method) or by adding sugar to wine vinegar (the commercial method). It also contains honey.

Creamy Caesar Dressing

Caesar salad has become a staple on restaurant menus everywhere. I do not get tired of Caesar salads because of all the variations in ingredients, such as grilled chicken, boiled shrimp, beef, or artichokes. My preference is for a Caesar salad to be sufficiently spicy, with well-blended garlic and anchovies in the dressing. This dressing is best prepared in a food processor or blender, so that the garlic and the anchovies are thoroughly pureed.

Serving size: 2 tablespoons

¼	cup mayonnaise
3	tablespoons fresh lemon juice (about one lemon)
1	teaspoon Dijon-style mustard
2	anchovy fillets, drained on a paper towel (you can refrigerate the remaining anchovies in their oil for another use, in a non-metal container)
2	cloves garlic, chopped
½	teaspoon Worcestershire sauce
4+	drops hot pepper sauce, such as Tabasco
4	tablespoons grated Parmesan cheese
¼	cup extra virgin olive oil
	Salt and freshly ground, black pepper

Add the mayonnaise, lemon juice, mustard, anchovies, garlic, and Worcestershire sauce to the blender or food processor and blend well. Add the hot pepper sauce and Parmesan cheese. Pulse to blend. Turn the machine on, and add olive oil in a steady stream. Taste and season with salt and pepper. Keep the dressing refrigerated.

Nutrition Analysis: 1 carb, 2 protein, 160 calories

Anchovies are rich in vitamin A, which is important for vision and bone growth. They are also high in calcium (also important for bone) and potassium, which is critical for your heart and other muscles to function properly.

Japanese Ginger Dressing

Serving size: 2 tablespoons

⅓   cup soy sauce
3   tablespoons lemon juice (about 1 lemon)
3   cloves garlic, pressed or minced
3   tablespoons minced fresh ginger
1   teaspoon Dijon-style mustard
2   teaspoons honey
     Freshly ground, black pepper (to your taste)
1   cup extra virgin olive oil

Add the soy sauce, lemon juice, garlic, ginger, mustard, honey, and black pepper to a blender or food processor. Puree these ingredients until the garlic and ginger are well incorporated and not chunky. While the machine is running, add the olive oil in a steady stream until it is well blended. Store the dressing in a glass jar in the refrigerator. Shake it or stir it well before using it. For recipes using this dressing, see Broccoli and Orange Salad on page 120 and Asian Salad with Snap Peas and Carrots on page 109.

Nutrition Analysis: 2 carbs, 1 protein, 171 calories

Ginger is not a root. Rather, ginger is the subterranean part of the stem. As an aid to digestion, it relieves gas and helps with nausea. Peel fresh ginger by scraping it with the back of a small spoon. Prepare only the portion that you need for any given recipe. You can refrigerate the remaining ginger root.

Sun-Dried Tomato and Anchovy Dressing

Sun-Dried Tomato and Anchovy Dressing is a thick dressing with many uses. It is excellent on grilled eggplant or roasted eggplant. You can try it on other vegetables or on salad greens. It is an excellent topping for hummus. Further, raw vegetables can be dipped in this dressing.

Serving size: 2 tablespoons

2	anchovies in oil, drained on a paper towel (you can refrigerate the remaining anchovies in their oil, for another use, in a non-metal container)
1	clove garlic, chopped
3	tablespoons capers, rinsed and drained
¼	cup sun-dried tomatoes in oil, chopped
½	cup extra virgin olive oil
2	tablespoons fresh lemon juice
2	teaspoons Dijon-style mustard
	Salt and freshly ground, black pepper

Place the anchovies, garlic, capers, and sun-dried tomatoes in a food processor and puree. Add the olive oil, lemon juice, and mustard. Pulse this mixture until it is well blended. Add salt and pepper to taste.

Nutrition Analysis: 1 carb, 0 protein, 133 calories

Give Anchovies a Chance! I know that many people will avoid recipes that include anchovies. But anchovies will allow you to achieve a savory, subtle flavor in certain recipes. So it is not about showcasing the anchovy! Buy small tins or jars of anchovies packed in oil. Rinse the anchovies in water before using, and store any remaining anchovies, in their oil, in a non-metallic container in the refrigerator, where they will keep for several days.

Mediterranean Chopped Salad
(no lettuce)

Traditional Greek salads such as Mediterranean Chopped Salad are not placed on top of lettuce. Rather, they are composed of chopped, fresh vegetables and fresh herbs. The fresh herbs bring so much flavor to this dish. It's imperative that you at least use fresh parsley, if not also fresh oregano and basil. If you get used to buying fresh herbs when you shop, you will find myriad ways to use them in your cooking.

This salad makes a wonderful accompaniment to grilled meat or fish. It should be prepared 1 hour before serving to let it have a chance to chill in the refrigerator.

4 servings

1	cup coarsely chopped, fresh, ripe tomatoes (or cherry tomatoes, halved)
1	cup peeled, diced cucumbers
4	artichoke hearts (canned), chopped
¼	cup thinly sliced, red onion
¼	cup pitted Kalamata olives, halved
1	clove garlic, minced
1	tablespoon chopped, fresh parsley
1	tablespoon chopped, fresh oregano
1	tablespoon chopped, fresh basil
	Grated peel ½ a lemon
1	tablespoon red-wine vinegar
1	tablespoon white-wine vinegar
¼	cup—plus 1 tablespoon—extra virgin olive oil
⅛	teaspoon crushed red pepper
	Salt and freshly ground, black pepper
½	cup feta cheese, crumbled

In a bowl, mix all of the ingredients together and refrigerate them for 1 hour before serving. Eat any leftovers the next day for lunch, packed in a pita, with cooked, grilled meat from last night's dinner.

Nutrition Analysis: 9 carbs, 4 protein, 257 calories

Tomato and Cucumber Salad

2 servings

1   medium tomato, chopped
½   medium cucumber, chopped (peeled if you prefer)
2   tablespoons chopped, fresh parsley
2   tablespoons extra virgin olive oil
       Salt and freshly ground, black pepper

In a bowl, mix the tomato, cucumber, parsley, and olive oil together. Add salt and pepper to taste. Serve as a side dish, in a small bowl. If you need to add carbs to your meal to reach 30 carbs, dip pieces of whole wheat pita into the olive oil at the bottom of your salad bowl.

Nutrition Analysis: 4 carbs, 1 protein, 137 calories (includes all of the olive oil)

Cucumbers are 95 percent water. Thus, when you eat cucumbers and other watery foods early in a meal (such as in a salad), they help you to feel fuller, faster. They are rich in magnesium and potassium, and so they may help to lower your blood pressure.

Avocado and Corn Salad with Lime Basil Vinaigrette

This Avocado and Corn Salad with Lime Basil Vinaigrette highlights fresh corn, and it is a real treat in the summer with corn straight from the farmers' market. Try to use corn that is so fresh that it has never been refrigerated. This salad has a lot of calories, but its calories are from two good sources: avocados and olive oil. Pair this salad with lean meat (such as chicken breast or fish) if you are counting calories for weight loss.

4 servings

Avocado and Corn Salad
1   avocado, chopped
1   ear fresh sweet corn, white or yellow
      Use any or all of these items as garnishes for this salad: vine-ripe tomatoes, fresh parsley, green onion, and red bell pepper or yellow bell pepper.

Lime Basil Vinaigrette
      Grated peel from ½ a lime
2   tablespoons fresh lime juice
1   teaspoon honey
3   tablespoons extra virgin olive oil
      Salt and freshly ground, black pepper
1   heaping tablespoon chopped, fresh basil

Prepare the vinaigrette in this manner. First, whisk the lime zest, lime juice, honey, salt, and pepper in a small bowl. Continue to whisk this mixture, and add olive oil in a steady stream to blend. Add the fresh basil. Husk and remove the silk from the corn, and wash the corn. Slice the corn off the cob, and place the corn in a small bowl. Add the chopped avocado. Pour this dressing over the vegetables, and mix gently to coat the vegetables.

Note that when this dressing is tasted alone, it is quite tart. But when the dressing is paired with the sweet corn, the tartness works well. Don't be tempted to add more honey.

Nutrition Analysis: 11 carbs, 2 protein, 197 calories

Cucumber and Yogurt Salad

2 servings

1	medium cucumber, peeled and thinly sliced
½	clove garlic, minced
	Freshly ground, black pepper
¼	cup Greek-style yogurt
2	tablespoons thinly sliced, fresh mint

In a bowl, mix the cucumbers, garlic, yogurt, and black pepper. Add the mint and stir to blend. Refrigerate the salad until it is ready to serve. This salad tastes best if you eat it on the same day that you make it.

Nutrition Analysis: 4 carbs, 3 protein, 53 calories

Asian Salad with Snap Peas and Carrots

2 servings

	Thinly sliced crisp lettuce and cabbage (use a mixture such as romaine lettuce, red cabbage, and Savoy or napa cabbage)
½	cup sugar snap peas, cut into bite-size pieces
1	medium carrot, shredded
¼	red bell pepper, cut into ⅛-inch slices, 1 to 2 inches long
1	teaspoon sesame seeds (or 1 tablespoon of chopped peanuts)
	Chopped, fresh cilantro or parsley (optional)
4	tablespoons Japanese Ginger Salad Dressing (page 103), refrigerated to be as cold as the salad

Combine all of the salad and vegetables in a medium bowl. Just before serving, add the Japanese Ginger Salad Dressing and toss to coat. Sprinkle the salad with sesame seeds or chopped peanuts and cilantro or parsley.

Nutrition Analysis: 9 carbs, 3 protein, 207 calories

If you add cooked chicken breast to this salad, then you have a hearty lunch salad!

Spinach and Mushroom Salad with Garlic Dressing

I found the basis for this recipe, Spinach and Mushroom Salad with Garlic Dressing, years ago in *Gourmet* magazine (which regrettably is no longer in publication). The original recipe included bacon and blue cheese croutons. I substituted the bacon and croutons with mushrooms and walnuts for a healthier, updated flavor profile. Garnish with blue cheese crumbles if you desire. This salad would make a delicious side to a simply grilled flank steak or other lean, red meat.

4 servings

4–6   cups fresh baby spinach, washed and dried
½   cup white mushrooms, wiped clean and thinly sliced
½   cup cherry tomatoes, halved
⅛   cup walnuts, coarsely chopped and toasted*

Garlic Dressing
1   clove garlic, chopped
½   teaspoon salt
¼   cup mayonnaise
2   tablespoons extra virgin olive oil
2   tablespoons red-wine vinegar
2   teaspoons honey

Make the dressing by first combining the garlic with the salt, mayonnaise, olive oil, vinegar, and honey; put them in a blender or a small food processor, and blend them until smooth.

In a medium bowl, toss the spinach leaves, sliced mushrooms, and tomatoes with the dressing. Top with chopped walnuts and serve.

Nutrition Analysis: 5 carbs, 1 protein, 193 calories

*Place chopped walnuts in a small skillet on the stove, over low heat. Stir the nuts occasionally and heat until fragrant. Immediately remove the walnuts from the hot pan, and cool them completely.

Marinated Sweet Peppers and Black Olive Salad

4 servings

¼	cup sliced, red bell pepper
¼	cup sliced, yellow bell pepper
¼	cup sliced, green bell pepper
¼	cup pitted, Kalamata olives, halved
½	small ripe tomato, coarsely chopped
4	tablespoons Sesame Dressing (see page 101)
4	tablespoons grated Parmesan cheese
	A mixed green salad

In a small bowl, mix the peppers and olives together. Coat them with Sesame Dressing. Marinate the peppers and olives for at least 1 hour (up to 4 hours).

Prepare a mixed green salad. Top the salad with the tomato and marinated vegetables. Add more Sesame Dressing if desired.

You can top each salad with 1 tablespoon of grated Parmesan.

Nutrition Analysis: 7 carbs, 2 protein, 206 calories (these numbers include 1 tablespoon of additional dressing per serving)

The difference between green olives and black olives is how long they are allowed to ripen. Green olives are picked earlier than black ones. Both types then go through a curing process to make them edible. Kalamata olives are named for the Greek town near where they are grown. When ripe, they are a dark-purple color.

Raw Zucchini with Lemon and Thyme

Use baby zucchini (or small, firm zucchini) for this mild, raw salad. If you slice the zucchini very thin (almost in ribbons), you can enjoy the zucchini's delicate flavor. To do this, first peel one side of the zucchini to provide a flat surface for stability on your cutting board. Or you can use a mandoline. Use the finger guard!

4 servings

3	small zucchini; trim the ends and peel one side
	Grated fresh lemon peel from ½ of a lemon
1	tablespoon fresh lemon juice
2	tablespoons extra virgin olive oil
2	teaspoons chopped, fresh thyme (you could also use mint or tarragon)
1–2	tablespoons grated Parmesan cheese
	Salt and freshly ground, black pepper

Place the flat side (the peeled side) of the zucchini on a cutting board and slice it very thinly into rounds. (Or, use a mandoline to slice long ribbons.) Place the slices into a medium bowl. Add the lemon peel, lemon juice, olive oil, salt, and pepper. Mix well. Add fresh thyme or other fresh herbs and stir the mixture to distribute the herbs. Allow the mixture to marinate while you prepare the rest of your meal. Top the zucchini with grated Parmesan cheese just before serving.

Nutrition Analysis: 3 carbs, 2 protein, 86 calories

> **A mandoline** is a handy slicer that can be set to a variety of widths to consistently slice fruits and vegetables. You can find this tool at just about any kitchen store or supermarket. Be sure to use the finger guard, because the blade is VERY sharp.

Italian Tomato Salad

The key to this salad is its simplicity. It uses vine-ripe, summer tomatoes. (Of course, vine-ripe summer tomatoes are nearly perfect without any accompaniments at all!)

2 servings

1	medium, vine-ripe tomato (heirloom are the most flavorful), sliced ¼-inch thick
2	teaspoons extra virgin olive oil
1	teaspoon balsamic vinegar
1	tablespoon thinly sliced, fresh basil
⅛	cup pine nuts (optional)

Place the tomato slices on two salad plates. Drizzle the slices with olive oil and balsamic vinegar. Top them with basil and pine nuts.

Nutrition Analysis: 5 carbs, 2 protein, 112 calories (these numbers include the pine nuts)

Quick Mexican Salsa

Okay, I know that salsa is not a salad. But it is fresh, and it's delicious on many dishes, including eggs (breakfast tacos), beans, and vegetables. Further, salsa makes a great dressing for fajita and taco salads. This recipe is just a guideline; you can mix all of these ingredients in a small bowl, and then you can add more of any ingredient to taste. Refrigerated, it lasts for 3 to 5 days.

Makes about 1 ⅛ cups (10 servings)

3	Roma (plum) tomatoes, diced
½	small, white onion, minced
½	fresh jalapeno or serano pepper, seeds and veins removed, minced
½	lime
¼	cup chopped, fresh cilantro (washed well, with its large stems removed)
	Dash ground cumin
	Dash garlic powder
	Salt and freshly ground, black pepper

Because cilantro stems are tender, they can be included in any dish that calls for cilantro. I like to cut off the large stem ends up to where the leaves begin. Then I chop the rest of the stem and use those pieces with the leaves.

Nutrition Analysis: per serving (2 tablespoons): 1 carb, 0 protein, 5 calories

Avocado Slaw

Part salad, part coleslaw, this crunchy and creamy salad is a great companion to fish and chicken. I make this slaw with any cabbage and crisp greens that I have on hand. Because it includes avocados, the slaw will not last overnight. Make only what you will eat immediately.

4 servings

4	cups various thinly sliced cabbage and crisp lettuce, such as napa cabbage (Chinese cabbage), red cabbage or radicchio, and escarole or romaine cores
2	green onions; thinly slice the parts that are green and white
1	avocado, cubed
¼	red bell pepper, thinly sliced (if you have it on hand)
2	tablespoons chopped, fresh cilantro (optional)

Dressing

2	tablespoons mayonnaise
2	tablespoons extra virgin olive oil
1	tablespoon fresh lime juice
⅛	teaspoon chili powder
	Salt and freshly ground, black pepper

Mix the salad ingredients together in a medium bowl. In a separate bowl, whisk the dressing ingredients together. Pour the dressing over the salad. Mix it to coat. Refrigerate this salad while you prepare the rest of your meal.

Nutrition Analysis: 6 carbs, 1 protein, 191 calories

Marinated Broccoli

You can use this recipe as the basis for Broccoli and Sun-dried Tomato Quinoa, on page 207.

2 servings

Marinade
1 ½	tablespoons extra virgin olive oil
1	tablespoon water
1	tablespoon white-wine vinegar
1 ½	teaspoons fresh lemon juice
1	teaspoon honey

Balance of Ingredients
1	clove garlic, minced
2	cups fresh broccoli florets (add the stems, chopped or sliced, if desired)
2	tablespoons chopped, red bell pepper
2	tablespoons chopped walnuts
¼	teaspoon salt
	Dash cayenne

Whisk the olive oil, water, vinegar, lemon juice, and honey in a small bowl. In a medium bowl, combine the broccoli, garlic, red pepper, walnuts, salt, and a sprinkle of cayenne. Pour the marinade over the broccoli mixture and stir well. Allow it to marinate at least 1 hour before serving.

Nutrition Analysis: 11 carbs, 4 protein, 183 calories

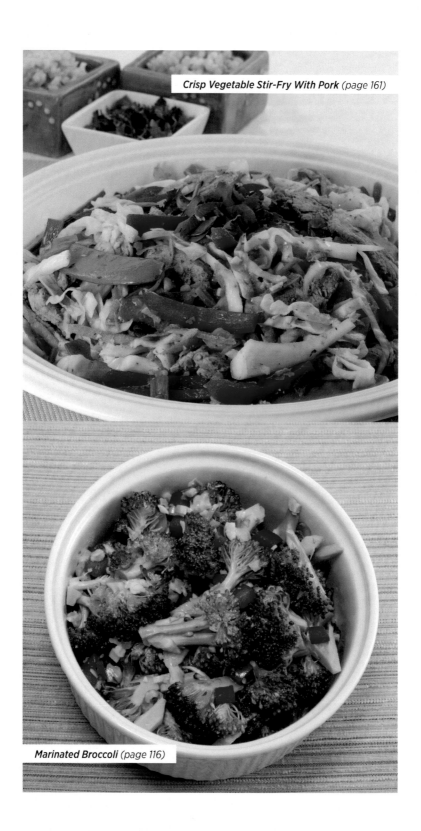

Crisp Vegetable Stir-Fry With Pork (page 161)

Marinated Broccoli (page 116)

Cool Cucumber and Cantaloupe Salad

Ripe cantaloupe, cucumber, and mint are cooling flavors in the heat of summer. Use this dish as a small side to bring your carb count up to 30 for a meal, or include it as an appetizer when you are entertaining (be sure to include a protein on the side).

8 servings; may be halved

1	medium, ripe cantaloupe; peel it, remove the seeds, and cube it
2	medium cucumbers, unpeeled, halved lengthwise and sliced ¼-inch thick (about 2½ cups)
	Grated peel from 1 lime
	Juice from 1 lime
1	tablespoon fresh, minced ginger
1	tablespoon honey
2	tablespoons chopped, fresh mint
	Pinch salt
	Pinch cayenne

Place the cantaloupe and cucumber into a large bowl. Add the lime peel, lime juice, ginger, and honey and gently mix well. Sprinkle with fresh mint, a pinch of salt, and a pinch of cayenne and mix just to distribute. This salad can be made up to 4 hours ahead of your meal. It tastes better if served at room temperature.

Nutrition Analysis: 10 carbs, 1 protein, 39 calories

Marinated Asparagus and Tuna Salad

Prepare the asparagus the night before and take this to work; your coworkers will be impressed. The marinated asparagus, topped only with the hard-boiled eggs (no salad, no tuna), also makes a great side dish for dinner (or part of an appetizer platter). You can double the recipe.

2 servings

1	recipe for Lemon Vinaigrette (page 99) with optional capers
¼	pound asparagus, trimmed, and stems peeled if you prefer (see the sidebar on how to do this)
1	tablespoon minced shallots
	Romaine lettuce (or other mix of fresh salad greens), washed and ready to eat
2	hard-boiled eggs
	Chopped, fresh parsley
	Salt and freshly ground, black pepper
1	(5-ounce) can high-quality tuna, drained

How to Prepare Asparagus

Asparagus ends become tough as they spend time in the market and your refrigerator. Some people snap off the ends where the asparagus naturally breaks. But I find that method a bit slow (working with one spear at a time) and wasteful. So simply line up your bunch of asparagus on a cutting board, cut off about once inch of the stems, and discard the ends. Now what about peeling the stems? I don't bother, unless I am making an elegant dish as part of a special meal.

Blanch the asparagus. Fill a 2- or 3-quart saucepan with water and bring the water to a boil. In the meantime, prepare an ice bath by filling a large bowl with ice water.

When the water is boiling, add a teaspoon of kosher salt, add the asparagus, and cook for 30 seconds. Drain the asparagus, and immediately submerge it in the ice water to stop the cooking process. Drain the asparagus and dry it on a clean kitchen towel or paper towel.

Add minced shallots to the Lemon Vinaigrette recipe. Cut the asparagus into 1-inch pieces (or keep the asparagus whole if you prefer). Place the asparagus into a dish just large enough to hold it, and pour enough vinaigrette over the asparagus to coat all of it. Allow it to marinate for several hours or overnight.

Prepare a salad of Romaine or other fresh greens. Peel and slice the hard-cooked eggs. Top the salad greens with asparagus, then the eggs, and then the tuna. Season with salt and black pepper. Add more vinaigrette to taste and top the salad with chopped parsley.

Nutrition Analysis: 3 carbs, 24 protein, 378 calories

Bring your carb count up by adding a whole wheat pita or a side of fruit.

Broccoli and Orange Salad

Broccoli, which is related to cabbage and Brussels sprouts, contains antioxidants. It is a good source of vitamin A, vitamin C, calcium, iron, and fiber. Broccoli has a lot of protein for a vegetable (almost 3 grams per cup). Today's broccoli casseroles and salads often smother this vegetable in fats (butter), starch (cracker crumbs), cheese sauce, and sugar. Here, in Broccoli and Orange Salad, is proposed a fresher way to enjoy the taste and health benefits of raw broccoli.

2 servings

2	cups broccoli florets and partial stems, sliced
1	medium carrot, peeled, shredded
2	tablespoons sweet onion, chopped
1	small orange, peeled and chopped
1	teaspoon sesame seeds
	Salt

Dressing

¼	cup of Japanese Ginger Salad Dressing (page 103)
1	tablespoon no-sugar-added peanut butter
⅛	teaspoon crushed red pepper

Mix the dressing ingredients. Prepare a salad and pour the dressing over the salad. Stir the salad to evenly coat. Serve immediately, or allow the salad to chill for several hours. This salad holds well overnight.

Nutrition Analysis: 19 carbs, 7 protein, 297 calories

Fresh Spinach with Oven-Roasted Cherry Tomatoes

This side dish coaxes extra flavor from winter tomatoes and pairs them with a healthy, winter green: fresh spinach.

2 to 4 servings

1	pint cherry or grape tomatoes, washed
1 ½	tablespoons extra virgin olive oil
	Salt and freshly ground, black pepper
	Fresh spinach, washed and dried
	Red onion
1	tablespoon balsamic vinegar
	Parmesan cheese, goat cheese, or blue cheese

Preheat oven to 325°F.

Toss the tomatoes in olive oil to coat, and season them with salt and pepper.

Lightly coat a baking sheet with olive oil. Place the tomatoes on the baking sheet, and place them in oven. Cook for about 1 hour, turning the tomatoes once or twice.

When the tomatoes are shriveled but not completely dry, take them out of the oven. Place the warm tomatoes in a small bowl, and drizzle them with 1 tablespoon of balsamic vinegar. Mix this well and allow it to cool.

Prepare a spinach salad. Wash and dry the spinach, and place it on a small plate or bowl. Top the salad with marinated tomatoes. Garnish it with thin slices of red onion and 1 tablespoon of grated Parmesan.

Nutrition Analysis:
2 large servings: 10 carbs, 4 protein, 152 calories
4 small servings: 5 carbs, 2 protein, 76 calories

Thai Meat-Patty Salad with Peanut Sauce

These meat patties are great for salads or burgers. For salads, shape them into meatballs. For sandwiches, make them into 4-ounce patties. You can portion and freeze the leftovers. I use a mixture of ground turkey (or chicken) and pork, but you can make these with only ground turkey (or ground chicken). You also can simply "scramble" the meat; add the spices and herbs, and serve the ground meat mixture on a salad or in lettuce wraps.

2 to 4 servings

1	pound ground turkey or chicken
1	pound ground pork
4	green onions, the green and white parts, thinly sliced
1	tablespoon ground coriander
1	clove garlic, minced
1	egg
1	tablespoon soy sauce
1	jalapeno, seeded, minced (or ½ teaspoon of crushed red pepper (optional)
½	cup chopped parsley
½	cup chopped cilantro
1	teaspoon toasted sesame oil
2	tablespoons extra virgin olive oil

In a large mixing bowl, mix all of the ingredients (except the sesame oil and olive oil). Shape into 1 ½ inch-diameter meatballs (about 1 ounce each), or 4-ounce patties.

Heat the sesame oil and olive oil in large skillet, over medium heat. If using meatballs, flatten those slightly to reduce the cooking time. Add these to the pan. Cook them on one side, about 2 to 3 minutes, to brown. Then turn them, and cook them another 3 minutes or until done.

The peanut sauce is used as a dressing for the salad or a sandwich.

Peanut Sauce
Makes 2 tablespoons (4 servings)

1	tablespoon peanut butter
1 ½	teaspoons tamari or soy sauce
1	teaspoon cider vinegar
1	teaspoon vegetable oil
½	teaspoon sesame oil
¼	teaspoon ground ginger
¼	teaspoon honey
	Dash cayenne
½	tablespoon chopped, fresh mint or cilantro (optional)

Place the peanut butter, tamari, vinegar, vegetable oil, sesame oil, ginger, and honey in a small bowl, and whisk these until creamy. Add cayenne to taste, and stir in mint or cilantro. Use on a salad or sandwich.

Nutrition Analysis:
10 servings (3 patties each): 1 carb, 16 protein, 227 calories
15 servings (2 patties each): 1 carb, 11 protein, 151 calories
Peanut Sauce: 1 carb, 1 protein, 4 calories

Serving Suggestions

- In cabbage or lettuce wraps.

- Over chopped salad of mixed greens and cabbage, sliced red bell pepper, and sugar snap peas.

- In half of a whole wheat pita, with shredded lettuce and cucumbers.

- Dress with peanut sauce or Annie's Goddess Dressing. Garnish with any of the following: fresh cilantro, mint, green onions, and/or fresh basil.

Turkey and Black Bean Taco Salad

You can use ground turkey, ground chicken, or shredded cooked chicken to make this variation on the taco salad. If you are not familiar with chipotle peppers, start with a small amount and test for heat level before adding more. You can buy small cans of chipotle peppers in adobo in the Mexican food section of your regular grocery store. Store the unused peppers, in their sauce, for later use, in a covered glass dish or plastic dish in your refrigerator.

4 to 6 servings

1	tablespoon extra virgin olive oil
1	pound ground turkey
1 ½	cups cooked, black beans (or one 15-ounce can, drained and rinsed)
½	small, white onion, chopped
1	clove garlic, minced
1	medium tomato, chopped
½	teaspoon dried oregano
1	chipotle pepper in adobo sauce, chopped
	Splash chicken broth or water
	Salt and freshly ground, black pepper
	Fresh lime juice
¼	cup fresh cilantro, chopped (optional)
	Salad greens

Heat the olive oil in a 10-inch skillet over medium heat. Add the ground turkey, and stir frequently to break up any lumps. Cook the turkey until it is just done but not browned.

Add the onion, and cook the turkey another 3 minutes, just until the onions begin to soften. Add the black beans, garlic, tomatoes, and oregano. Mix it well. Add chipotle peppers and enough broth (or water) to keep the mixture moist.

Heat the mixture through and taste for hotness; add more chipotle peppers if desired. Add salt and freshly ground, black pepper to taste. Squeeze fresh lime juice into the mixture to taste (start with ¼ lime), and add cilantro if desired.

Remove the mixture from the heat and allow it to cool slightly before adding it to your salad.

Prepare the salad greens, and top the greens with this mixture of meat and beans. No dressing is required. But you can add vegetables and garnish as you would for your favorite taco salad: a bit of cheese, avocado, fresh tomato, olives, sour cream, and so on, and count the carbs, protein, and calories of these items.

Nutrition Analysis: 19 carbs, 26 protein, 300 calories

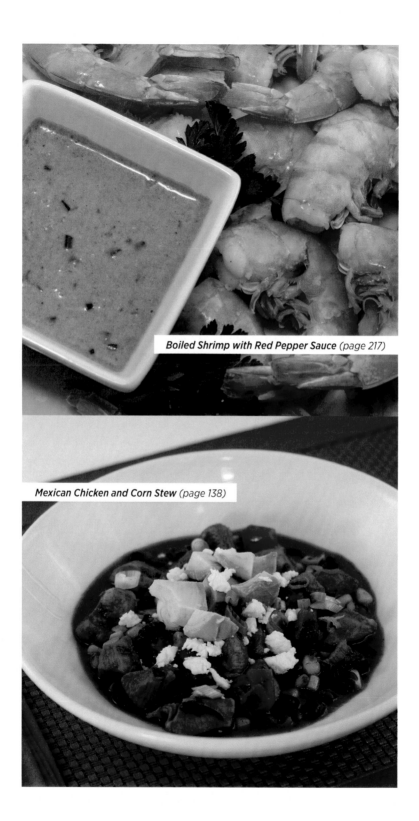

Boiled Shrimp with Red Pepper Sauce (page 217)

Mexican Chicken and Corn Stew (page 138)

CHAPTER 12

Satisfying Soups and Stews

Soups and stews make wonderful one-pot meals for busy households. To me, nothing is as nourishing and nurturing as a steaming bowl of "dinner." Plus, leftovers are often even better the next day and make great lunches.

I rarely follow a recipe for soup because I use vegetables that I have on hand. To these I add protein, a seasoning of herbs or spices, and then garnish the soup with fresh greens, fresh herbs, maybe hot sauce, perhaps avocado, or a grate of Parmesan.

I use homemade chicken broth any time I have it. I buy whole chickens and roast them. Then I use the backs, wings, and carcasses from the roasted chickens to make broth. After a batch is made, I freeze it. My pantry also includes store-bought organic chicken broth and vegetable broth, too.

Don't be shy about modifying recipes to suit your taste. If you don't like mushrooms, for example, leave them out. If you do like mushrooms, add more.

The soup recipes in this book will give you ideas about what flavors work well together. Because I am counting grams of carbs now, I modified some of my old standbys (like black bean chili) to include more protein and fewer carbs.

The following tips will help you to get the most from your soups and stews.

- Sauté your "flavor-base" vegetables, such as onions, carrots, celery, bell peppers, leeks, and mushrooms. You can cook these vegetables in olive oil before adding any broth. Cooking these items first intensifies their flavor.

- Add chopped, fresh greens (such as kale, spinach, Swiss chard, and so forth) to soups just a few minutes before serving for added nutrition and color.

- Toss yellow squash, zucchini, chopped cabbage, or tomatoes into almost any soup. These mild vegetables won't add many carbs or affect the overall flavor of the soup.

- Use previously cooked meat (such as roast chicken, steak, pot roast, or meatballs) for a quick soup.

- Rather than boil your soups and stews, simmer them. Even meat cooked in liquid will get tough if overcooked.

- Heat the broth before adding it to the soup, for a quicker cooking time.

- Thaw frozen vegetables before adding them to your soups.

- Use pureed or mashed cooked beans (or canned beans) as a thickener. Be sure to count the carbs.

- Add small portions of lentils, beans, barley, or brown rice to your soups if you need to add carbs.

- Add fresh herbs toward the end of the cooking time, and sprinkle fresh herbs as a garnish to really bring out that flavor.

- Accompany your soup with a small side salad if you have not already had your "salad a day."

Beef and Vegetable Soup with Paprika and Marjoram

I created this soup one day while emptying my vegetable drawer into the soup pot. That's the beauty of soup. I always have onions, celery, and carrots on hand. Marjoram is a nice herb to use with soups and with egg dishes, so I keep that on hand as well. Marjoram is similar to oregano, but milder. The cooking time is longer for this soup than for other soups, to allow the beef to become tender and the marrow to release from the bone into the soup.

4 to 6 servings

2–2 ½ pounds beef shank with bone
1   tablespoon extra virgin olive oil
1   cup chopped onion
1   cup chopped celery
1   cup chopped carrots
2   bay leaves
4–6   cups vegetable broth

8 cups of mixed vegetables, such as
  • tomatoes, chopped
  • cabbage, chopped
  • broccoli florets
  • mushrooms, cleaned and sliced
  • green beans, cut into 1-inch pieces

1 ½   tablespoons sweet paprika
¾   teaspoon dried marjoram
      Dash cayenne
      Salt and freshly ground, black pepper

Season the beef shank with salt and pepper. Heat the olive oil in a large (6 to 8 quart) pot, over medium-high heat. Add the beef shank, and brown on both sides (so cook it about 2 minutes per side). Remove the beef shank from the pan. Add the onion, celery, and carrots to the pan, and cook 2 minutes, stirring to remove any brown bits from the bottom of the pan. Add 4 cups of vegetable broth and bay leaves, and return beef shank to the pot. Bring the food to a boil. Reduce the heat, and simmer the soup for 60 minutes until the beef is tender and the bone is clean.

Remove the beef and bone from the pot. Allow the beef to cool, and cut it into bite size pieces. Discard the bone.

Add the mixed vegetables, and add additional 1 to 2 cups of vegetable broth if desired. Bring the soup to a boil, then reduce the heat to a simmer. Add sweet paprika, dried marjoram, cayenne, salt, and black pepper to taste. Cook the soup 20 minutes, and then serve it.

Nutrition Analysis: 21 carbs, 25 protein, 239 calories

Thanksgiving Soup

Sweet potato and broccoli star in this bright soup. Use leftover roasted holiday turkey or rotisserie chicken for a great flavor.

6 servings

2	tablespoons extra virgin olive oil
3	cups cooked turkey (light and dark meat)
1	small onion, chopped
1	cup chopped celery
1	clove garlic, minced
2	cups broccoli florets, the stems separated and chopped
2	medium sweet potatoes, peeled and cubed (about 2 cups total)
1 ½	cups black beans, cooked or 1 can (15 ounce), rinsed and drained
6	cups chicken broth
1	bay leaf
1	teaspoon dried thyme
½	teaspoon dried oregano
⅛	teaspoon ground allspice (or ground nutmeg)
	Hot pepper sauce, such as Tabasco

Heat the olive oil in a large saucepan, over medium-high heat. Add the onion, celery, garlic, and broccoli stems. Sauté those ingredients until they are softened (about 5 minutes), stirring often.

Add the chicken broth, turkey, broccoli florets, sweet potatoes, black beans, bay leaf, thyme, oregano, and allspice. Bring the soup to a simmer, and cook it until the sweet potatoes are tender, about 10 to 12 minutes. Serve with hot pepper sauce on the side.

Nutrition Analysis: 23 carbs, 27 protein, 268 calories

Sweet potatoes have low glycemic index; for their size, they have fewer carbohydrates than regular potatoes. So pound for pound, when you eat sweet potatoes, not only are you eating fewer carbohydrates, but also the carbohydrates that you are eating are better for you.

Chicken and Squash Chili

My sister gave me this basic recipe years ago, and I have seen variations of it printed in many cookbooks and magazines (and on a can of Bush's Beans) since then. In this version, I incorporate vegetables in the chili and use roast chicken for a more savory dish. In this recipe, some of the beans are for the chili, but some are saved to use as a thickener.

6 servings

3	cups cooked chicken (roast chicken, if you have it)
1	tablespoon extra virgin olive oil
1	medium onion, chopped
2	cloves garlic, minced
3	cups chicken broth
3	cups cooked cannellini beans; or 2 cans (15 ounce), drained and rinsed—set 1 cup aside
2	small, yellow squash (or zucchini), chopped (about 2 cups)
2 ½	teaspoons ground cumin
1	(4-ounce) can chopped, green chilies
1 ½	teaspoons dried oregano
	Salt and freshly ground, black pepper to taste
	Chopped cilantro for a garnish
	Other optional garnishes: 1 tablespoon of shredded, Cheddar cheese, chopped avocado, or pickled jalapenos.

Heat the olive oil in large sauce pan, over medium heat. Then add the onion, and cook it until it is soft (about 5 minutes). Add the garlic, and cook the onion for 2 minutes more. Add broth and cooked chicken.

Reserve one cup of the rinsed beans to use as a thickener. Add the remaining beans to the chili. Also, add the yellow squash or zucchini. Stir in cumin, oregano, and green chilies. Reduce the heat to low, and simmer uncovered for 25 minutes.

Puree or mash the remaining beans; you may need to add a little broth or water, if necessary, to create a smooth paste. Add the paste to the chili. Add salt and pepper to taste. Add more cumin and oregano to taste. Simmer the chili for 15 minutes more.

You can garnish the chili with chopped, fresh cilantro. If you like, you can also garnish the chili with 1 tablespoon of shredded Cheddar cheese, chopped avocado, or pickled jalapenos.

Nutrition Analysis: 26 carbs, 28 protein, 282 calories

Creamy Chicken and Barley Soup

I use barley in this soup rather than noodles, because barley has a lower glycemic index (it has a lot of fiber); but you could substitute whole wheat pasta instead. Note that barley has a long cooking time (50 to 60 minutes); but you can soak barley overnight, and if you do so, then it will cook in 15 minutes.* So plan ahead for this soup, and you'll have dinner on the table in no time. Mushroom, barley, lemon, and heavy cream are a great combination. You can double the amount of mushrooms to 8 ounces for a more pronounced flavor (I do).

4 to 6 servings

1	pound boneless, skinless chicken breast, cut into bite-size pieces (or 2 ½ cups cooked chicken, cut into bite-size pieces)
2	tablespoons extra virgin olive oil
1	small onion, chopped
1	medium carrot, chopped
1	celery rib, chopped
4	ounces white mushrooms, cleaned and sliced
4	cups chicken broth
½	cups pearled barley, presoaked and uncooked
1	teaspoon dried thyme
1 ½	tablespoons fresh lemon juice
½	cup heavy cream
	Salt and freshly ground, black pepper

Heat olive oil in a large saucepan. Add the onions, carrots, celery, and mushrooms. Sauté the mixture until the vegetables are almost soft (about 7 minutes). Add the chicken and chicken broth, and bring the soup to a simmer. Skim off any foam that rises. Add barley, thyme, and lemon juice, and then reduce the heat to medium low. Simmer the soup, uncovered, for 20 minutes.

Add heavy cream, and increase the heat slightly to bring the soup back to a simmer. Add salt and black pepper to taste.

*If you do not presoak the barley, then combine 1 ½ cups water with ½ cup barley in a medium saucepan. Bring the barley to a boil; cover it and cook it for 50 minutes. Drain it, and add barley to the soup with the thyme and lemon juice. Cook the soup for 5 minutes before adding the heavy cream.

Nutrition Analysis: 26 carbs, 31 protein, 378 calories. Why does this soup have more calories than most of the other soups? Heavy cream!

Lean Beef and Bean Chili

Great beef chili is based on the building blocks of quality meat, sweet vegetables, and not too much tomato. This recipe is easily doubled, but do not double the cumin and chili powder at once—add those two spices in small doses until you get the flavor and heat level you like. (When I barely feel the chili powder at the back of my throat, I know I have added enough.) You should chop the onions and bell peppers very small so that they almost disappear into the chili. In this recipe, some of the beans are used for the chili, and some are used as a thickener.

6 servings

1 ½ pounds lean, red meat, such as ground sirloin or bison (or sirloin steak cut into bite size pieces)
1   tablespoon extra virgin olive oil
1 ½ cups finely chopped onion
2   cloves garlic, minced or pressed
½   cup finely chopped, red bell pepper
½   cup finely chopped, green bell pepper
1   tablespoon ground cumin
1   tablespoon sweet paprika
2   tablespoons chili powder*
3   cups cooked, black beans; or dark-red kidney beans; or 2 cans (15 ounce) of either type of beans, drained and rinsed—set aside 1 cup
1   cup chopped tomatoes
2   cups vegetable broth
1   teaspoon dried oregano
     Salt and freshly ground, black pepper
     Other garnish options: chopped avocado or shredded cheese.

Heat the olive oil in a large saucepan, over medium heat. Add the onions and peppers, and sauté, stirring often until the onions and peppers are soft and almost caramelized (about 10 minutes).

Add the garlic and ground or chopped beef. Cook the chili, stirring often, for about 3–5 minutes.

Add cumin, paprika, and chili powder, and mix well. Add the beans (except for the reserved beans), tomatoes, and broth. Bring the chili to a boil, then reduce the heat to medium low, and simmer the chili for 20 minutes, uncovered.

Mash or puree the reserved beans. If necessary, you can add a bit of water or broth. Mix the mashed beans into the chili. Add the oregano, salt, and pepper, and simmer the chili for another 10 minutes.

Garnish the meal with your choice of chopped, white onions, chopped tomatoes, chopped avocado, or shredded cheese.

Nutrition Analysis: 28 carbs, 34 protein, 332 calories

*Optional: Replace the chili powder with canned chipotle peppers in adobo, which are smoked jalapeno peppers in a vinegar-based sauce. Start with ½ to 1 whole pepper. Chop the pepper and add it to the chili when you would add the chili powder. Taste the mixture and add more chipotle pepper if desired. Save the remaining canned chipotle peppers, for another use, in a non-metallic container in the refrigerator.

Curry Chicken and Lentil Stew

Serve this stew for dinner with a simple, mixed-green salad. Or you can portion it to take to work for a hearty lunch.

4 servings; may be doubled

12	ounces boneless, skinless, chicken breast, cubed
2	tablespoons extra virgin olive oil
1	medium onion, diced
½	cup finely chopped celery (about 1 large rib)
½	cup finely chopped carrots
2	cups kale, with the stems removed; wash it and chop it
2	cloves garlic, minced
2 ½	tablespoons sweet curry powder
1	teaspoon garam masala
4	cups (32 ounces) chicken broth
¾	cup dried, green lentils
½	teaspoon salt and freshly ground pepper
	Hot pepper sauce, such as Tabasco

Heat the olive oil in a large saucepan, over medium heat. Add the onion, celery, and carrots. Cook this mixture, stirring often, about 7 minutes. Add the chicken, and cook the stew, stirring it, for 3 to 5 minutes. Add the garlic, curry powder, garam masala, salt, and pepper; mix the stew well. Add the lentils and chicken stock, and stir.

Bring the stew to a boil, then reduce the heat enough to allow a brisk simmer. Cover the saucepan partially, and simmer the stew for 25 to 30 minutes (until the lentils are tender, but not mushy).

Add the kale. Return the stew to a simmer, and cook it for another 5 minutes.

Serve the stew with hot pepper sauce on the side.

Nutrition Analysis: 28 carbs, 33 protein, 344 calories

Earthy Leek and Mushroom Soup

In this recipe, leeks, celery, carrots, mushrooms, and cabbage meld together for a velvety, earthy soup. Don't be tempted to substitute onions for the leeks.

4 servings

3	cups cooked chicken
1	bunch leeks (2 or 3 leeks); use the white and light green parts only, washed and sliced crosswise*
2	ribs celery, with the leaves, finely chopped
3	carrots, peeled and sliced
4	ounces mushrooms, cleaned and sliced
2	cloves garlic, minced
2	tablespoons extra virgin olive oil
6	cups chicken broth
¼	small head cabbage, thinly sliced (3–4 cups total)
1	dried bay leaf
½	teaspoon dried oregano
½	teaspoon dried thyme
	Dash allspice
	Dash cloves
	Dash cayenne
	Salt and freshly ground, black pepper

Heat the 2 tablespoons of olive oil in large saucepan, over medium heat. Add the leeks, celery, mushrooms, and garlic. Cook until the leeks are soft and almost caramelized (about 10 to 15 minutes). Stir the mixture occasionally.

Add the broth, carrots, cabbage, and the dried bay leaf. Bring the soup to a boil, reduce the heat, and simmer it until the carrots are tender (about 15 minutes).

Add the chicken, oregano, thyme, allspice, cloves, and cayenne. Season it with salt and freshly ground, black pepper. Cook the soup 5 minutes more, to thoroughly heat the chicken before serving.

Nutrition Analysis: 21 carbs, 35 protein, 367 calories

*Leeks are similar to onions, but milder. They are sold by the bunch; so whether the bunch has two or three leeks, I use the entire bunch. Leeks are sandy, so wash them carefully to remove all that sand before using them. For a soup such as this one, simply remove the dark-green, upper portion of the leek, slice the leeks crosswise, and discard the hairy end of the bulb. Immerse the slices into a bowl of cold water. Swish the slices to rinse them, drain them through a colander, and repeat.

Mexican Chicken and Corn Stew

4 servings

1	pound boneless, skinless, chicken breast, cubed
1	tablespoon flour
2	tablespoons chili powder
2	teaspoons ground cumin
½	teaspoon garlic powder
½	teaspoon salt
	Freshly ground, black pepper
1	cup fresh or frozen corn kernels, thawed
1 ½	cups cooked black beans, or 1 (15 ounce) can drained and rinsed
1	cup chicken broth
1	cup chopped, fresh tomatoes
⅓	cup chopped cilantro
2	tablespoons canola oil
	Optional garnishes: feta cheese, or shredded Cheddar cheese and chopped avocado

For this recipe, use a plastic container with a lid that is big enough to hold the chicken. In that container, combine the flour, chili powder, cumin, garlic powder, salt, and black pepper. Whisk the mixture to blend it well. Add the chicken, then cover the container with its lid and shake it to coat all chicken pieces evenly.

Heat canola oil in large, deep skillet or saucepan, over medium heat. Add the chicken and cook it until it browns. Stir it often. Be careful not to cook it too long, or you may burn the spices. Even if the chicken is not completely cooked yet, do not worry because the chicken will cook more in the stew.

Add the corn, black beans, chicken broth, and tomatoes. Bring the food to a simmer, then reduce the heat to medium low. Simmer the meal uncovered for 12 to 14 minutes until the stew is slightly thickened. Stir it occasionally.

Add the chopped cilantro, and mix it well. Taste, and add more salt if needed. Garnish with feta cheese or shredded Cheddar cheese and chopped avocado. Or you can make a small side salad of romaine lettuce, avocado, extra virgin olive oil, and a squeeze of lime juice.

Nutrition Analysis: 26 carbs, 34 protein, 324 calories

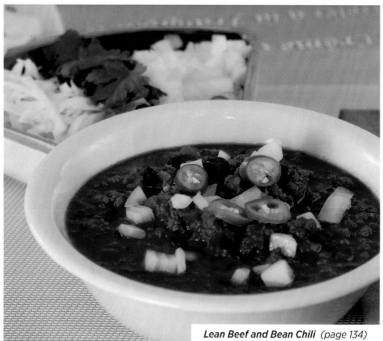

Lean Beef and Bean Chili (page 134)

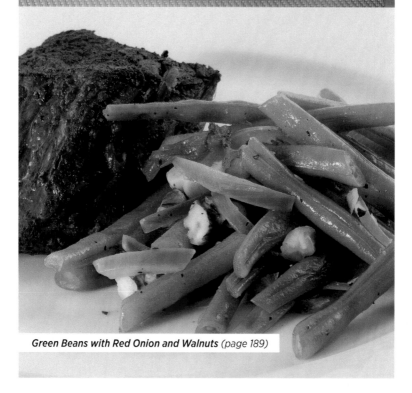

Green Beans with Red Onion and Walnuts (page 189)

CHAPTER 13

Lean Meat, Lean Body

Wellness 100 balances protein and carbohydrates for health and weight management. Under the guidelines of Wellness 100, you should eat at least 70 grams of protein per day (not per meal, per day). Dr. French recommends lean meats as an important source of protein, along with fish (see Chapter 14 on fish dishes).

On the Wellness 100 program, you may be eating less meat per meal. But also on this diet, you may be eating as much or more meat than you formerly would eat in a whole day. (If you previously ate cereal for breakfast and pizza for lunch.) Plan to cook an extra portion at night, so that you can use the leftovers for breakfast and lunch. It won't take any more time to do this task; but over the next few days, by doing so, you will save a lot of time (and decisions about "what's for lunch?"). Get in the habit of portioning leftovers to freeze. Label your freezer items for quick reference. Keep a roll of masking tape in your kitchen. Secure a small piece to your wrapped item or container, and use a Sharpie to write the contents and date.

Lean meats are those that have less than 10 grams of fat, 4.5 grams or less of saturated fat, and less than 95 grams of cholesterol per 3.5-ounce serving. You can use Table 13.1, "Lean Meat Choices," to help you make great meals.

Table 13.1
Lean Meat Choices

Cut of Meat	Saturated Fat (grams)	Total Fat (grams)
Top round roast and steak	1.9	5.4
Bottom round roast and steak	2	5.7
Top sirloin steak	2.2	5.7
95% lean ground beef	2.7	6
Round steak	2.2	6.2
Chuck shoulder pot roast	2.1	6.7
Flank steak	3	7.7
Tenderloin roast and steak, i.e., T-bone, filet mignon, New York strip, and porterhouse	3.2	8.3

Cut of Meat	Saturated Fat (grams)	Total Fat (grams)
T-bone steak	3.5	9.6
Veal	2.4	6.2
Chicken breast (skinless)	1	3.6
Ground chicken breast	0	1
Turkey breast (skinless)	0.2	0.7
Ground turkey breast, 93% lean	2.2	7.1
Pork loin/chop	0.7	2.3
Pork sirloin roast	2.8	9.3
Ham	2.3	5.8
Flounder	0.4	1.5
Mahi-mahi	0.3	0.9
Halibut	0.4	2.9
Sea bass	0.7	2.6
Grouper	0.3	1.3
Salmon (wild, not farm raised)	1	6.3
Tilapia	0.9	2.7
Shrimp	0.3	1.1
Lobster	0	0
Crab	0.1	0.6
Lamb chop	3.5	9.6
Rabbit	2.4	8
Venison	1.2	3.2
Pheasant	1.1	3.3
Bison steak	1.9	5
Elk	1.5	5

Oven-Roasted and Braised Meat

Oven roasting and braising offer advantages for cooking large cuts of meat. You can achieve great flavor with little effort: season or marinate the meat, and then it's mostly hands off, which allows you to prepare the side dishes. You can plan to use your oven for double duty, and you can roast vegetables or bake gratins at the same time as the meat is cooking. You can enjoy a comforting Sunday dinner and have enough leftovers for another meal or to use as a base for lunch salads, soups, and stews during the work week.

Roast Chicken

The best advice I can give you for a simple roast chicken is to start with an organic free-range chicken; it tastes better, and it's better for you. Buy a 4- to 5-pound chicken.

1	whole organic chicken, 4 to 5 pounds
2	large carrots, cut into 2-inch pieces
2	celery ribs, cut into 2-inch pieces
1	small onion, peeled and quartered, layers separated
½	cup water
	Salt and freshly ground, black pepper
	Extra virgin olive oil

Preheat the oven to 400°F. Remove the neck and organs from the cavity; rinse it inside and out, and pat it dry with a paper towel. I like to cut a few slits through each side of the backbone (parallel to the backbone, underneath the bird) to allow the juices from inside the bird to gradually drip out of the chicken. I don't like to have any pink juice flowing out of the cavity when I carve the bird. Season the inside with salt and pepper, and place a quartered lemon and/or a few sprigs of fresh thyme inside the chicken—or not!

Place the prepared carrots, celery, and onion on the bottom of a shallow roasting pan, and add about ½ cup of water to the pan. Season these vegetables with salt and pepper. Place the chicken on the vegetables breast side up–there is no need to truss the chicken, but it does help to tuck the wing tips behind the wings. Drizzle extra virgin olive oil over the top side of the bird, and rub the skin for a uniform coating. Season the breast and sides of the bird with more salt and freshly ground pepper.

Place the chicken in the hot oven. Cook for 20 minutes, and reduce the oven temperature to 350°F. Add more water to the pan as needed, and cook it for 1 hour to 1 hour and 15 minutes. Test for doneness by piercing the bird in the thickest part of the thigh. If the juices run clear, then the bird is done. Or you can use an instant-read thermometer and place it in the same spot until it reads 165°F to 170°F.

If the skin of the chicken starts to get too brown before the chicken reaches 165°F, tent it with foil and continue cooking it. Remove it from the oven, tent it with foil, and allow the chicken to rest for 10 minutes before carving it. Its temperature should rise another 5°F after it is removed from the oven.

Use leftover roast chicken to top a hearty dinner salad. Pull the chicken off the bones. Then heat 2 teaspoons of olive oil in a nonstick skillet, add the chicken to briefly warm it, and season it with salt, pepper, and dried oregano. Place the warmed chicken on top of your favorite salad of mixed greens, vegetables, and vinaigrette. Note that there are other recipes in this book in which to use any remaining pulled chicken.

Nutrition Analysis:
3.5 ounces of cooked meat (light), no skin, has 0 carbs, 31 protein, 165 calories
3.5 ounces of cooked meat (dark), no skin, has 0 carbs, 27 protein, 205 calories

Roast Pork Loin

This recipe will be using a marinade, so you may want to do the marinating overnight or at least for a few hours. Use one pork loin. Choose one that is 3 to 4 pounds, boneless, and center-cut. If the pork loin is not trimmed, then remove the silver skin and trim off the large pieces of fat. But retain a thin layer of fat (about ⅛-inch thick) on one side of the roast.

1	boneless pork loin, 3 to 4 pounds
1	Lemon-Rosemary Marinade (page 159)

Heat the oven to 450°F. Prepare the Lemon-Rosemary Marinade on page 159. Slather a thick coating of marinade on the pork loin (you can marinate the pork loin for several hours or overnight for a more pronounced lemon and rosemary flavor). Place the pork fat-side-up on a roasting rack in a shallow roasting pan. Cook it for 10 minutes, then reduce the oven to 325°F and continue cooking it for 40 to 50 minutes more. Test it with an instant-read thermometer. Cook it until the pork reaches 140°F to 145°F. Remove it from the oven and tent it with foil. Let it rest for 10 minutes before slicing. (Its temperature should rise about 5°F while it rests.)

In 2011, the U.S. Department of Agriculture lowered its recommended safe-cooking temperature for pork to 145°F from 160°F. Please note that at 145°F, pork may still look a little pink, but that is okay.

Nutrition Analysis: 3.5 ounces cooked meat has 0 carbs, 28 protein, 207 calories

Pot Roast with Sweet Onions

1	boneless beef chuck roast or rump roast, 3 to 4 pounds
3	large yellow onions, cut in half and sliced about ¼-inch thick
1	12-ounce beer (lager or dark beer, not light beer)*
2	bay leaves
3	cloves garlic, chopped
½	teaspoon dried thyme
1	tablespoon red-wine vinegar
	Salt and freshly ground, black pepper
	Extra virgin olive oil
	You might need water or a light beef broth.

*Substitute light beef broth (beef broth and water) for the beer, if you do not want to use beer.

Heat the oven to 325°F (or you can use a crock pot set on low heat after you add the ingredients). Caramelize the onions. Heat 2 tablespoons of olive oil in a large frying pan, over medium heat. Add onions to the pan and stir to coat evenly. Cover the pan, reduce the heat to medium low, and cook it for about 20 minutes, stirring occasionally to make sure they are not browning. Continue cooking until the onions are soft and golden in color (about 10 more minutes).

Pat the roast dry, and season it all over with salt and pepper. Heat 1 tablespoon of olive oil in large, wide, heavy pot, over medium-high heat. Brown the beef on all sides, and transfer it to a plate.

Transfer the onions to a Dutch oven, a roasting pan with a lid, or a crock pot. Add the bay leaves, garlic, beer, red-wine vinegar, about 1 teaspoon of salt, and ½ teaspoon of black pepper. Stir it to mix. Place the beef roast on top; add water or light beef broth (if necessary) to almost cover the roast. Cover the pan and cook the roast at 325°F for about 3 hours (check for doneness after 2 ½ hours). If you are cooking the roast in a crock pot, set it to low and cook for 6 to 8 hours.

Remove the roast from the liquid, and use a slotted spoon to remove the onions. Serve the roast with a spoonful of caramelized onions.

Nutrition Analysis: 3 ounces cooked meat has 0 carbs, 28 protein, 180 calories

Roast Bone-in Turkey Breast
(Half-Breast or Whole Breast)

	Half-breast or whole breast of turkey, bone-in
2	tablespoons slightly softened butter
1	teaspoon dried sage
¼	teaspoon dried thyme
½	teaspoon salt
¼	teaspoon freshly ground, black pepper

Heat the oven to 350°F. Prepare a compound sage–butter: Mix 2 tablespoons of slightly softened butter with 1 teaspoon of dried sage, ¼ teaspoon of dried thyme, ½ teaspoon of salt, and ¼ teaspoon of freshly ground, black pepper.

Rinse the turkey breast, and pat it dry with paper towels. Spray a shallow roasting pan and rack with nonstick cooking spray. Place the turkey breast on the rack. Loosen the skin from the meat, but do not remove the skin. Rub the breast under the skin with the compound butter. Drizzle the top of the skin with about 1 teaspoon of extra virgin olive oil. Bake the turkey for about 20 minutes per pound until an instant-read thermometer reads 160°F. Remove the turkey from the oven, and tent it with foil. Allow it to rest for 10 minutes before slicing.

Use the turkey meat for sandwiches and salads. Also, you can substitute cooked turkey for chicken in any of the recipes in this book that call for cooked chicken.

Nutrition Analysis: 3.5 ounces cooked meat has 0 carbs, 30 protein, 135 calories

Slow-Roasted Pork Shoulder
(Pork Butt)

Pork shoulder, also known as "pork butt," is a fatty cut of pork. When slow-roasted, it becomes tender and flavorful. Use a boneless pork shoulder (as in this recipe) for a shorter cooking time. Pork butt does not meet the program's criteria for lean meat (except for its cholesterol level). Thus, be sure to trim the exterior fat from the shoulder before cooking the roast to eliminate excess saturated fat.

Also, remove the roast from the drippings before slicing it (or shredding it) and storing.

1	boneless pork butt, exterior fat trimmed off, 5 to 7 pounds
3	tablespoons extra virgin olive oil
1	tablespoon white-wine vinegar, or another mild, white vinegar
2	tablespoons grated orange zest
3	cloves garlic, minced
2	teaspoons ground ginger
1	tablespoon dry mustard
1	tablespoon crushed red pepper
2	teaspoons salt
1	teaspoon freshly ground, black pepper

Pork butt must be cooked to a higher temperature than lean cuts of pork (such as loin), in order to break down the fat and collagen (protein fibers) in the meat.

Preheat the oven to 450°'F. Combine the olive oil, vinegar, and all the remaining seasonings. Set the pork butt in a large roasting pan, and spread the rub over all sides of the pork butt. Roast it for 25 minutes. Reduce the oven to 325°F, and roast the meat for 3 ½ to 4 ½ hours until the roast reaches 185°F. (The pork will shred easily with a fork.)

Transfer the meat to a platter or cutting board, and tent it with foil. Let it rest for 15 minutes before serving. Discard the drippings (the fat).

Nutrition Analysis: 3 ounces cooked meat has 0 carbs, 21 protein, 227 calories

Pecan-Crusted Chicken Breast

A live-aboard sailor friend gave me this recipe years ago when we lived next to each other at a marina in Texas. Living in close proximity to your neighbors (as you do on a sailboat) means that you get to smell what's for dinner all around you! I like this simple recipe so much that I even rotated it on my "specials board" at my café.

The high calorie count is due to the pecan crust. Serve this chicken with steamed broccoli or simple green beans and half of one baked sweet potato.

4 servings

4	small boneless, skinless chicken breast halves (1 to 1 ¼ pounds total)
1 or 2	limes, for juicing
	Salt and freshly ground, black pepper
¾	cup finely chopped pecans
½	cup plain bread crumbs or Panko
¼	teaspoon dried basil
⅛	teaspoon cayenne
2	tablespoons extra virgin olive oil, plus more if needed

Preheat the oven to 400°F.

Rinse the chicken, and dry it on paper towels. Cover the chicken pieces with plastic wrap, and use a meat mallet or rolling pin to gently "pound" the chicken to a uniform thickness of about ½ inch. (Hit the thickest part of the chicken first, and then move outward toward the edges.)

Make the pecan mixture. Put the pecans and bread crumbs into a small bowl. Crumble the dried basil between your fingers into the bowl, and add the cayenne. Mix it well.

Squeeze the lime juice into a pie pan, and season the lime juice with salt and pepper. Pour the olive oil into a separate, large, oven-proof glass casserole dish or pie plate, and coat the bottom. Dredge the chicken in the seasoned lime juice, and then coat the chicken with the pecan mixture. Place the chicken in the casserole dish. Drizzle another teaspoon of olive oil on the top of the coated chicken pieces.

Place the casserole dish with the chicken into the oven, and bake it for 7 minutes. Turn the chicken pieces over, and drizzle them with more olive oil, if needed. Bake the chicken for another 5 to 8 minutes or until the chicken is cooked through.

Nutrition Analysis: 10 carbs, 34 protein, 402 calories

Curry Ground Beef with Peas

This meal can be served over a small portion of couscous. Or it can be served with whole wheat pita and steamed cauliflower (the garam masala is a great companion to cauliflower). The leftovers are delicious the next day for lunch, as well.

4 servings

1	pound lean, ground beef
4	cloves garlic, minced
2	tablespoons minced fresh ginger, divided in half
4	teaspoons garam masala, divided in half
3	teaspoons sweet curry powder
⅛ to ¼	teaspoon cayenne
1	medium onion, chopped
½	teaspoon salt
	Freshly ground, black pepper
2	medium-ripe tomatoes, coarsely chopped
½	cup Greek yogurt, optional
1	cup frozen peas, thawed
⅓	cup cilantro, chopped
2	tablespoons extra virgin olive oil

Heat the olive oil in a large, deep skillet over medium-high heat. Add the garlic, half of the garam masala (1 tablespoon), half of the minced ginger (1 tablespoon), curry powder, and cayenne. Begin to cook, stirring it, just to release the fragrance of the spices (about 1 minute).

Add the onions, and reduce the heat to medium; cook until the food is softened (about 5 minutes). Add the ground beef, salt, and pepper, and cook it through, stirring often to break up any lumps. Taste for seasoning, and add more cayenne, curry, and salt to taste.

Add the peas and the tomatoes, and cook it through (another 5 to 7 minutes).

Add the remaining ginger, the remaining garam masala, yogurt, and cilantro. Stir it, and serve.

Nutrition Analysis: 13 carbs, 30 protein, 320 calories, based on adding yogurt

Curry powder is a mixture of several spices, usually including coriander, turmeric, cumin, fenugreek, and red pepper. Garam masala is also a mixture of spices, usually including black and white peppercorns, Malabar leaves, cloves, mace blades, star anise, nutmeg, coriander, cardamom, and cumin.

Friday-Night Fajitas

You will be marinating this recipe's beef or chicken overnight, so start on Thursday with the marinade.

In no time at all, it's Friday night! So you want to relax after a busy work week, and you're looking for a treat. Skip the pizza! Let these fajitas be your Friday-night fun meal. Top them with sautéed peppers and onions, sliced avocado, fresh salsa, and sour cream, and serve them with a side of beans. Remember to go easy on the tortillas.

8 servings

Fajita Marinade

¼	cup soy sauce
¼	cup canola oil
2	teaspoons sesame oil
2	tablespoons honey
2	tablespoons cider vinegar
½	teaspoon ground ginger
1	teaspoon garlic powder
2	tablespoons finely chopped, green pepper
2	pounds boneless, skinless chicken breasts or flank steak

Whisk all of the marinade ingredients together. Place the meat in a shallow container or a plastic, sealable bag. Pour the marinade over the meat, and refrigerate it 8 hours or overnight.

When you are ready to cook the meat, place a wire rack on a rimmed baking sheet. The wire rack will allow the meat to drain. Remove the meat from the marinade, and place it on the rack. Allow it to reach room temperature (about 30 minutes). Cook the meat in a skillet or on a medium-hot grill.

Nutrition Analysis:
3 ounces of cooked flank steak has 0 carbs, 24 protein, 173 calories
3.5 ounces of cooked chicken breast has 0 carbs, 31 protein, 165 calories

Greek Burgers

Serve these burgers on sandwich thins or in a whole wheat pita with lettuce, mustard, and sliced red onion.

4 servings

1	pound lean, ground beef
½	cup finely chopped, red onion
1	clove garlic, minced
1	egg, beaten
¾	teaspoon dried thyme
¼	teaspoon dried oregano
½	teaspoon salt
	Freshly ground, black pepper
½	cup feta cheese, crumbled

Lean, ground meat (and grass-fed meat) benefits from being cooked at a medium-to-low heat. Grilling should not equate to charring, burning, or scorching!

Place the ground beef into a medium bowl. Add the onion, garlic, egg, thyme, oregano, salt, and pepper. Using your hands, mix the ingredients together. After it is well mixed, add the feta cheese, and mix gently.

Portion the beef into four (4-ounce) patties.

Grill or cook them in a large skillet, over medium heat.

Nutrition Analysis: (for meat patties only): 3 carbs, 30 protein, 243 calories

Skillet Chicken, Three Ways

These savory chicken dishes don't require much work but do deliver a lot of flavor. Once you get all the ingredients in the pan, it is hands-off while it simmers. Serve with a simple side salad, and enjoy a piece of fruit for dessert to get the carbs that you need.

Start with a whole chicken, or buy the chicken already cut up. I use a whole, organic chicken because it's cheaper to buy the whole bird than parts.

1. Sweet Red Peppers, Tomatoes, and Fennel

1	whole, small, organic chicken (about 3 ½ pounds), cut into pieces, breasts cut in half (crosswise)
¼	cup olive oil
½	large, red bell pepper, sliced ¼-inch thick
3	ripe Roma tomatoes, coarsely chopped
½	cup fresh fennel bulb, sliced ¼-inch thick
¼	cup pitted Kalamata olives
1	clove garlic, minced
½	cup dry white wine
2	tablespoons of chopped, fresh oregano

Rinse and pat dry the chicken pieces. Season them with salt and freshly ground pepper. In a large skillet with deep sides, heat the olive oil over medium-high heat. Add the chicken pieces to brown, and do not over-crowd the pan. (Brown in two batches if necessary.) Brown on all sides (8 to 10 minutes total). Remove the chicken from the pan. Reduce the heat to medium, and remove all but one tablespoon of oil from the pan.

Add the peppers, tomatoes, fennel, olives, and garlic to the skillet. Return all the chicken pieces to the skillet, and add white wine. Bring the food to a boil. Reduce the heat to medium low, and partially cover it. Simmer it about 40 minutes (until chicken is tender and cooked through). Add fresh oregano, and serve.

Nutrition Analysis: 8 carbs, 30 protein, 322 calories

2. Creamy Lemon and Artichokes

1	whole small organic chicken (about 3 ½ pounds), cut into pieces, breasts cut in half crosswise
¼	cup olive oil
2	anchovy fillets, drained
2	cloves garlic, minced
2	lemons, juiced
½	cup chicken stock
1	(8.5-ounce) can whole artichoke hearts, drained, with the artichokes cut in half
¼	cup heavy cream
1 ½	teaspoons fresh thyme (or ½ teaspoon dried thyme)
	Chopped, fresh parsley

Rinse and pat dry the chicken pieces. Season them with salt and freshly ground pepper. In a large skillet with deep sides, heat the olive oil over medium-high heat. Add the chicken pieces to brown, and do not over-crowd the pan. (Brown in two batches if necessary.) Brown on all sides (8 to 10 minutes total). Remove the chicken from the pan. Reduce the heat to medium, and remove all but one tablespoon of oil from the pan.

Add the anchovies, and stir as they quickly melt into the oil. Add the garlic, and return all of the chicken pieces to the pan. Add the lemon juice and chicken broth. Bring it to a boil, and then reduce the heat to medium low, and partially cover it. Simmer it for 30 minutes. Add the artichoke hearts and thyme to the pan, and cook it for another 10 minutes (or until chicken is tender and cooked through).

Add the heavy cream, and blend well, bringing the cream sauce to a simmer. As soon as the mixture simmers, then turn the heat off, and add chopped parsley to garnish.

Nutrition Analysis: 7 carbs, 31 protein, 325 calories

3. Mushrooms, Onions, and Tarragon

1   whole, small, organic chicken (about 3 ½ pounds), cut into pieces, breasts
          cut in half crosswise
       salt and freshly ground, black pepper
¼   cup olive oil
8   ounces white mushrooms, cleaned, the tough stems removed, and sliced
1   large sweet onion, halved and sliced ¼-inch thick
1   clove garlic, minced
¼   cup dry, white wine
⅓   cup chicken stock
2   tablespoons butter
1   tablespoon chopped, fresh tarragon (or 1 teaspoon dried tarragon)

Rinse and pat dry the chicken pieces. Season them with salt and freshly ground pepper. In a large skillet with deep sides, heat the olive oil over medium-high heat. Add the chicken pieces to brown, and do not over-crowd the pan. (Brown in two batches if necessary.) Brown on all sides (8 to 10 minutes total). Remove the chicken from the pan. Reduce the heat to medium, and remove all but one tablespoon of oil from the pan.

Add the mushrooms, onion, and garlic to the pan, and stir. Return all of the chicken to the pan. Add the white wine and chicken broth. Bring it to a boil, then reduce the heat to medium low, and partially cover it. Simmer it until the chicken is tender and cooked through (about 40 minutes).

Remove the chicken from the pan, and turn off the heat. Add the butter and fresh tarragon. Taste the sauce, and add more salt and tarragon if needed.

Nutrition Analysis: 7 carbs, 31 protein, 339 calories

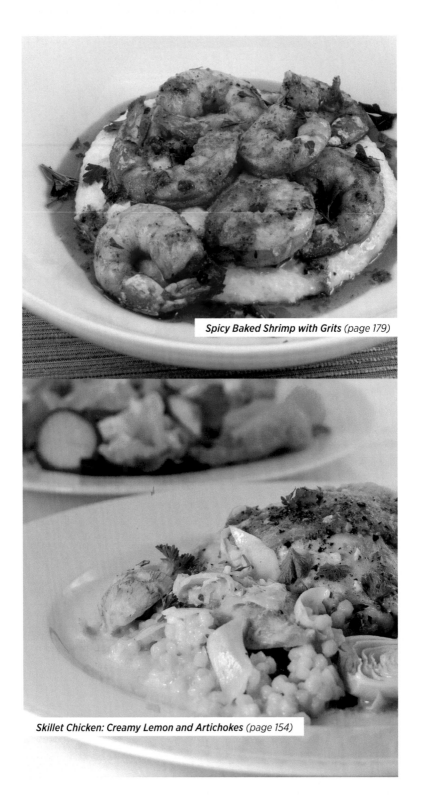

Spicy Baked Shrimp with Grits (page 179)

Skillet Chicken: Creamy Lemon and Artichokes (page 154)

Grilled Steak with Chimichurri Sauce

Chimichurri sauce is prevalent in South America, specifically in Argentina. It is basically a pesto made of parsley, olive oil, garlic, and crushed red pepper that is served alongside grilled meat. Use any cut of lean steak that you prefer for this recipe. I prefer flank steak.

This recipe makes more sauce than you will need for dinner. Refrigerate the remaining chimichurri sauce to use with other simply prepared meat or vegetables, or on eggs. You can even use it as a salad dressing, with a meat-topped salad the next day.

Serves 4

Chimichurri Sauce
Makes about 1 ½ cups

¼	cup red-wine vinegar (or white-wine vinegar)
2	tablespoons lemon juice
3	cloves garlic, chopped
1	teaspoon salt
	Freshly ground, black pepper
½	teaspoon crushed red pepper
4	cups fresh parsley
1 ½	cups fresh cilantro
¾	cup extra virgin olive oil
20	ounces (or more for more servings) flank steak, or other preferred steak
	Salt and freshly ground, black pepper
	Paprika

Combine the vinegar, lemon juice, garlic, salt, pepper, and crushed red pepper in a blender (or food processor) and blend it until the garlic is finely chopped. Add the olive oil and blend well. Add parsley and cilantro, and then pulse—stopping to scrape down the sides of blender or processor—until the sauce is almost smooth.

Prepare a grill or broiler. Season the steak on both sides with salt, pepper, and paprika. Cook the meat to desired doneness. Cover it loosely with foil, and allow it to rest for 5 minutes before slicing it and serving. Serve it with chimichurri sauce.

Grilled lamb chops or lamb loin chops would also work well with this recipe. A nice addition would be to add ½ cup of fresh mint to the chimichurri sauce.

Here's a tip for using parsley and cilantro. Cut off the bare stem ends of the parsley and cilantro bunches to the point where the leaves begin (about where the wire or rubber band starts). Wash the herbs in cold water to remove any sand. Drain well—or spin them dry in your salad spinner. The remaining stems are tender and can be included in the chimichurri sauce.

Nutrition Analysis: 3 ounces of cooked meat served with 2 tablespoons chimichurri has 2 carbs, 25 protein, 303 calories

Pork Chops and Sour Cream Cabbage

Add a side salad or another hot vegetable to this dish, and you've got real comfort food!

4 servings

4	small pork chops or 2 large pork chops (weighing 1 to 1 ¼ pounds total)
1	tablespoon extra virgin olive oil
	Salt and freshly ground, black pepper
1	(8 ounce) package white mushrooms, tough stems removed, cleaned, and thickly sliced
2	cloves garlic, minced
3	tablespoons fig-infused vinegar or pear-infused vinegar (Alessi brand is found in most supermarkets)
5	cups chopped, green cabbage or Savoy cabbage (1-inch pieces)
¼	teaspoon ground ginger
¼	cup + 2 tablespoons sour cream

Season the pork chops with salt and black pepper. Using a 10- to 12-inch skillet with a lid, heat olive oil over a medium-high heat. Add the pork chops, and brown the chops on both sides (1 to 2 minutes per side). Remove the pork chops from the pan, and reduce heat to medium low.

Add the fig-infused vinegar and mushrooms, and stir to coat. Cook the mushrooms for about 2 minutes to allow some of the vinegar to evaporate. Add the garlic, cabbage, ground ginger, and additional salt and pepper. Stir well, and cook it for about 5 minutes. Stir the cabbage mixture again, and place the pork chops on top, adding any juices from the meat back to the pan. Cover it, and cook approximately 10 minutes more, or until the pork chops are cooked through.

Remove the pork chops from the pan, and keep them warm. Add the sour cream to the cabbage, and mix well to form a creamy sauce. Spoon the cabbage mixture on plates, and top it with a pork chop.

Nutrition Analysis: 13 carbs, 31 protein, 296 calories

Lemon-Rosemary Marinade

This recipe uses a marinade, so you will want to refrigerate the meat in the marinade for a few hours or overnight. If you like rosemary, you will like this marinade on many types of meat for roasting or grilling. Meats that go with this marinade include pork (pork tenderloin, loin, and chops), chicken (pieces or boneless, skinless breasts), lamb chops, or steak. (It is great on kebabs, too!) You can grill or roast extra meat to add to a Greek salad the next day.

Marinade
- 2   cloves garlic, minced
- 3   tablespoons minced onion
- 2   tablespoons chopped, fresh rosemary
- 2   tablespoons fresh lemon juice
- 2   tablespoons white balsamic vinegar
- ¼   cup extra virgin olive oil
- ½   teaspoon freshly ground, black pepper

Mix the garlic, onions, rosemary, lemon juice, vinegar, olive oil, and black pepper in a small bowl, and whisk these ingredients until they are well blended. Place your choice of meat in a small glass container or a plastic sealable bag. Add the marinade, and coat the meat. Refrigerate the meat for a few hours or overnight. Remove the meat from the marinade, and grill it or roast it.

You can also try this marinade for grilled portobello mushrooms; but in that case, marinate the mushrooms for only 30 minutes.

Nutrition Analysis: See Appendix B (page 223) for meat and poultry nutrition data.

Sirloin Marinated in Red Wine

This recipe uses a marinade, so you will want to marinate the meat for 24 hours. Use a thick cut of sirloin (1 inch to 1 ½ inches).

4 servings

16 to 20 ounces thick sirloin steak
½   cup port wine or a full-bodied red wine
½   cup soy sauce
¼   cup olive oil
½   teaspoon black pepper
½   teaspoon dried thyme
¼ to ½ teaspoon Tabasco Sauce
1   clove garlic, minced
1   bay leaf

Mix all of the marinade ingredients in a small bowl. Place the sirloin and marinade in a shallow container with a lid. Cover and refrigerate it for 24 hours.

Prepare the grill to be at medium heat. Remove the steak from marinade, and grill it to desired doneness. Cover it loosely with foil, and allow the steak to rest for 5 minutes before slicing; then serve.

Nutrition Analysis (per 3.5 ounces of cooked meat): 0 carbs, 29 protein, 212 calories

Sirloin is considered a lean cut of beef, according to its saturated and total fat content. Be sure to trim off any visible fat to keep the calories from saturated fat as low as possible.

Grilling to excess is not healthy over the long term. By "excess," I mean grilling too often, or grilling at too high of a heat, or grilling meat until it is too well done. It is best to grill occasionally, using medium heat. Grill the meat to medium well, at most.

Crisp Vegetable Stir-Fry with Chicken, Beef, Pork, or Shrimp

This recipe is inspired by a recipe for simple, fried spring rolls. Crisp vegetables, fresh ginger, and lean meat make this dish light. Serve it over a small portion of brown rice, or supplement your carbs after the meal with fresh fruit (such as pineapple, plums, or peaches).

Stir-frying does not require high heat. Lean meat, thinly sliced, and sliced vegetables can quickly overcook. Thus use medium heat to medium-high heat, at most. First you will be making the sauce. Then you will continue with the recipe.

4 servings

16   ounces lean meat: pork, beef, or chicken, thinly sliced; or shrimp, peeled
         and deveined
      Freshly ground, black pepper
1   tablespoon soy sauce
½   cup chicken broth
2   tablespoons sherry vinegar or rice vinegar
1   teaspoon cornstarch

NOTE: Make the sauce before continuing (see the following directions).

2   cloves garlic, minced
1   tablespoon minced fresh ginger, plus 1 extra teaspoon set aside
½   small, Savoy cabbage or green cabbage, thinly sliced (4 cups), kept
         separate from other vegetables
4   green onions, green and white parts, sliced diagonally about ¼-inch thick
2   cups mixed additional vegetables (choose one or all):
         • Snow peas, tips and strings removed
         • Mushrooms, cleaned and sliced
         • Red bell pepper, sliced ¼-inch thick
2   medium carrots, peeled and shredded, set aside
      Chopped, fresh cilantro
1   tablespoon + 2 teaspoons extra virgin olive oil
2   teaspoons toasted sesame oil

Prepare the meat. Generously season it with freshly ground, black pepper. Set it aside in a small bowl.

Whisk the soy sauce, chicken broth, vinegar, and cornstarch in a small bowl. Add 3 to 4 tablespoons of the sauce mixture to the meat; stir to coat. Allow the food to marinate while you prepare the vegetables.

Heat 1 tablespoon of extra virgin olive oil in a large skillet, over medium heat. Add the meat and a pinch of the fresh, minced garlic and ginger to the pan. Cook the meat until done, but not dry. Transfer it from the pan to a large platter.

Add about 1 teaspoon of sesame oil to the pan, with 1 teaspoon of olive oil, and then add the cabbage, garlic, and 1 tablespoon of ginger. Cook the food, stirring constantly, about 2 minutes. (The cabbage will be wilted, but still crunchy.) Transfer this mixture to the platter with the meat.

Add the remaining 1 teaspoon of sesame oil and 1 teaspoon of olive oil to pan. Add the green onions and mixed vegetables; stirring this constantly, cook it another 2 minutes.

Add the sauce to the pan with the vegetables, and cook it about 1 minute, until slightly thickened.

Turn off the heat. Add the cabbage and meat from the platter back to the pan, along with the shredded carrots and the remaining 1 teaspoon of fresh, minced ginger. Season it with salt, and stir just to combine.

Pour the stir-fry onto the platter, and garnish it with chopped cilantro.

Nutrition Analysis (averaged for beef, chicken, or pork): 11 carbs, 28 protein, 303 calories

Koftas (Meat Patties) with Yogurt Sauce

Middle Eastern koftas are often pressed onto a skewer and grilled (or made into meatballs). I like meatballs and burgers of all kinds, and I could devote an entire chapter to "meatballs around the world." For ease of cooking, I make them into small patties to eat as a main course. That's also an ideal size to stuff in a pita for lunch.

4 servings

1	pound lean, ground beef or lamb*
1	teaspoon cinnamon
1	teaspoon curry
½	teaspoon cumin
2	cloves garlic, minced
½	cup minced, red onion
½	teaspoon freshly ground, black pepper
½	teaspoon salt
	Extra virgin olive oil

Place the ground beef in a large bowl, and add the remaining ingredients. Use your hands to thoroughly mix the spices, garlic, and onion into the beef.

Shape into 2-inch patties that are about 1-inch thick. You will then have eight (2-ounce) patties. Refrigerate the patties while you make the yogurt sauce.

½	cup Greek yogurt
1	clove garlic, minced
½	cup chopped, peeled cucumber
2	tablespoons chopped, red onion
1	tablespoon chopped, fresh mint

Mix all the ingredients together.

Heat 1 tablespoon of extra virgin olive oil in a large skillet, over medium heat. Add the meat patties, and cook them on one side for 5 minutes. Turn the patties, and cook them another 5 minutes (or until they are cooked through). An alternative method would be to heat a grill to low heat, and then grill the meat patties. Dress these with yogurt sauce.

Appetizer Variation: You can make these into 1 ½-inch meatballs. Cook the meatballs in a skillet with olive oil, and then serve them as an appetizer.

Nutrition Analysis: (including sauce): 6 carbs, 32 protein, 286 calories

*If you use ground lamb instead of beef, consider adding 1 tablespoon of chopped, fresh mint to the meat mixture, along with the other spices.

Mojo Marinade for Meat and Fish

This marinade is adapted from two Cuban marinades: an adobo marinade and a mojo criollo (a cooked version). Both of those Cuban marinades are based on garlic and citrus. Double the following recipe for whole chicken or pork roasts (in which case, count on marinating for several hours or overnight).

3	cloves garlic, minced
½	teaspoon ground cumin
½	teaspoon dried oregano
2	tablespoons chopped, fresh cilantro or parsley
3	tablespoons fresh lime juice
2	tablespoons extra virgin olive oil
	Salt and freshly ground, black pepper
	Boneless, skinless chicken breast (or firm fish)

Marinate the meat or fish for 30 minutes to 1 hour. You can use boneless, skinless chicken breast, pork, or firm fish. Grill the food over a medium to low heat.

If you are using this marinade with a whole chicken or pork roast, allow the meat to marinate several hours or overnight.

Nutrition Analysis: See Appendix B (page 223) for meat and poultry nutrition data.

Ginger and Soy Glazed Chicken

Briefly simmering a simple sauce creates a glaze that continues to thicken and turn slightly sticky in the oven after it is applied to the chicken. You may choose to use boneless, skinless chicken breasts in this recipe. If you do, it will take less time to cook.

6 to 8 servings

1 whole chicken, cut up (or equivalent, in pieces)

Ginger and Soy Glaze

4	cloves garlic, minced
¼	cup soy sauce
2	tablespoons toasted sesame oil
1	tablespoon fresh ginger, minced
2	tablespoons honey
2	tablespoons rice vinegar
½	teaspoon crushed red pepper
1	teaspoon mustard powder
2	tablespoons tomato paste
½	teaspoon freshly ground, black pepper

Preheat the oven to 375°F. Whisk all of the glaze ingredients together in a small saucepan. Place the pan over medium heat, and bring the glaze to a simmer. Reduce the heat to medium low, and simmer for 7 more minutes. Put the glaze aside to cool slightly.

Apply a nonstick cooking spray to an oven-proof baking dish or rimmed baking sheet. Whether you use a dish or a sheet, make sure you choose one large enough to hold the chicken pieces in a single layer. Place the chicken pieces on the prepared pan, skin-side up. Spoon all of the glaze over the chicken to coat it evenly. Bake the chicken for 40 to 50 minutes, or until it is done.

Nutrition Analysis: 3.5 ounces of cooked chicken (light and dark meat, no skin) has 0 carbs, 29 protein, 185 calories

Steak, Pork, or Chicken with Wine and Mushroom Sauce

The tarragon in this sauce is particularly nice with steak. You can substitute dry, white wine for the red wine if you desire a lighter sauce for meats such as chicken or pork. If you don't keep wine, use chicken broth and a squeeze of lemon juice for tartness.

2 servings; may be doubled

4	ounces white or portobello mushrooms, cleaned, tough stems removed, and sliced ⅛-inch thick (measures about 2 cups)
2	teaspoons olive oil
1	teaspoon butter
1	tablespoon minced onions or shallots
	Salt and freshly ground, black pepper
⅓	cup dry, red wine (or dry, white wine—see the previous introductory description)
1	teaspoon chopped, fresh tarragon or parsley
2	tablespoons heavy cream

Heat the olive oil and butter in a small saucepan, over medium heat. Add mushrooms, and stir to coat. Add the onions (or shallots) and dash of salt and pepper. Cook it until the mushrooms are soft and have released their moisture. Add the wine, and bring it to a simmer. Simmer the food until the wine is nearly gone (about 10 minutes). Add the tarragon and heavy cream; continue simmering it until it is slightly thick. Season it with more salt and pepper, if desired.

Turn leftover steak into another nice meal with this sauce. Slice the steak into strips about ¼-inch thick. Prepare the red wine mushroom sauce as described previously, and then add the steak to the sauce (in order to reheat the steak).

Nutrition Analysis: 5 carbs, 3 protein, 162 calories
With 3.5 ounces cooked beef: 5 carbs, 32 protein, 374 calories

This simple, delicious sauce may not contribute many carbs to your meal, but it does pack some calories and saturated fat due to the heavy cream and butter. It's a good idea as part of this meal to serve simple, steamed or roasted vegetables and a side salad.

Turkey and Italian Sausage Meat Sauce

Although I rarely eat pasta, I occasionally crave "spaghetti sauce." Italian sausage has more saturated fat than you should eat on a regular basis. But if sausage is paired with lean, ground turkey breast, it makes a delicious protein-rich dinner. Serve this meat sauce on sautéed eggplant and zucchini. You can also use spaghetti squash instead of pasta; if so, start baking the squash before you make the sauce (see the sidebar on the next page). Another idea is to make a small portion of pasta and sautéed vegetables.

4 servings

8	ounces ground turkey breast
8	ounces (about 2 links) sweet Italian sausage, casing removed
1	tablespoon extra virgin olive oil
1	cup finely chopped onions
½	cup finely chopped, green bell pepper
½	cup finely chopped, red bell pepper
4	ounces white mushrooms, sliced (about 1 ¼ cups)
3	cloves garlic, minced
2	(15 ounce) cans diced tomatoes; drain one can, but do not drain the other
2 ½	teaspoons dried basil
¾	teaspoon dried oregano
¼	teaspoon crushed red pepper
½	teaspoon salt
	Freshly ground, black pepper

Cook the turkey and Italian sausage in a 2-quart saucepan on medium heat, stirring often to break up any lumps. Reduce the heat if necessary to avoid browning the meat. When the Italian sausage is cooked through, spoon off any fat from the pan, and transfer the meat mixture to a bowl.

Add one tablespoon of olive oil to the saucepan, and add the onions, green pepper, red pepper, mushrooms, and garlic. Stir. Cook over medium heat until the vegetables are soft, stirring often (about 5 minutes).

Return the meat mixture to the pan with the vegetables, and mix it well.

Add the 2 cans of diced tomatoes (1 can drained and 1 can undrained). Add the basil, oregano, crushed red pepper, salt, and pepper. Bring the sauce to a simmer, and reduce the heat. Cook it, uncovered, for about 30 minutes. Stir it occasionally. The sauce will thicken as it cooks.

Nutrition Analysis: 15 carbs, 24 protein, 325 calories

Have you tried spaghetti squash?
It is a healthy substitute for pasta. Spaghetti squash takes about 45 minutes to bake, so be sure to start baking the squash before you make the sauce. Preheat the oven to 375°F. Cut the spaghetti squash in half, lengthwise. Remove the seeds. Brush the cut sides with olive oil and sprinkle the squash with salt and pepper. Place the squash on a rimmed baking sheet; cut sides down, and cover it with foil. Bake it until it feels tender to you when you pierce it with a fork (about 45 minutes). Allow it to cool slightly, then use a fork to remove the strands of spaghetti squash from each shell half.

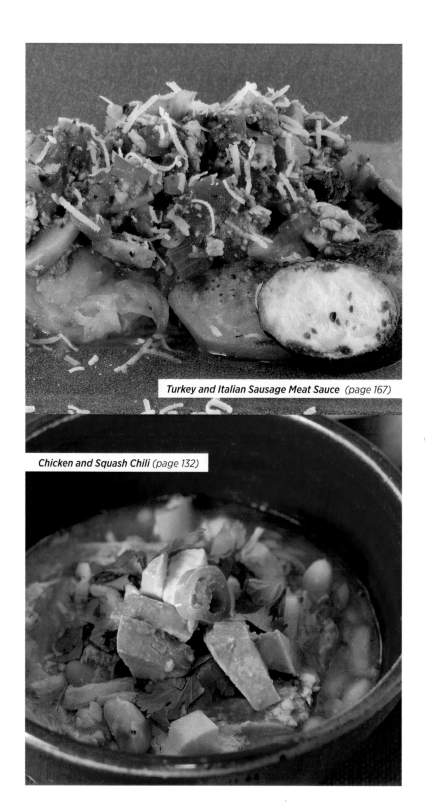

Turkey and Italian Sausage Meat Sauce (page 167)

Chicken and Squash Chili (page 132)

CHAPTER 14

Fish Twice a Week

High-quality, fresh fish does not require much in the way of preparation. On the other hand, you don't have to settle for just baked fish with a sprinkle of lemon pepper in order to avail yourself of healthful seafood. The following recipes for fish and shrimp will give you meals that you can conquer any evening, so that you can enjoy eating fish twice a week (or more). You can buy different types of fish to try in the various recipes. I buy a variety of wild-caught, saltwater fish, depending on what is available and how it is priced. (I prefer snapper, grouper, halibut, cod, amber jack, mahi-mahi, and salmon.)

How many times have you heard, "Fresh fish should not smell fishy"? As a generalization, this advice is true. Fish at the market should not smell fishy; it should smell like the sea. Sometimes when I buy fish, the grocer places it in a plastic bag; and when I open the bag the next day, it does smell a bit fishy. Don't worry if this happens to you. Just rinse the fish, pat it dry with a paper towel, and the fish should no longer have that odor. But any time fish smells very pungent or like ammonia, that odor is a sign of spoilage, and you should not buy it. If you just purchased it, then take the fish back to your supermarket for a refund.

Store your wrapped fish on a bed of ice in the coldest part of your refrigerator (usually the bottom shelf toward the back of the refrigerator) to maintain the best quality. If you are not going to cook the fresh fish the same day as your purchase (or the next day), then freeze it for use in the near future (within 1 month is best). Wrap it well in plastic wrap. Label and date the package, and freeze it. If you routinely freeze your fish, ask the market if they have the fish that you want already frozen. Today much seafood and shellfish arrives at the market frozen. It is thawed for display at the seafood counter.

To prepare fish for cooking, first remove any bones. Then you will want to remove the skin. To do so, first place the fish on a flat cutting surface. Then hold the tip of the narrow end of the fish (the tail end). Slide a thin, sharp knife under the meat just in front of your fingers, flattening the knife next to the skin, and making sure not to slice through the skin. Continue to hold the fish and to move the knife under the fillet next to the skin. Rinse the fish in cold water, and dry it on paper towels to remove excess moisture.

Although fresh fish is always better than canned fish, remember that adding high-quality canned tuna to lunch salads during the week is another way to incorporate seafood into your diet. Smoked fish should be consumed only occasionally or not at all.

Seared Fish with Tomato Cream Sauce

2   (4- to 5-ounce) fillets of firm, white fish (such as amber jack or halibut), skin removed
     Fresh lemon
     Salt and freshly ground, black pepper
     Sweet Hungarian paprika

Tomato Cream Sauce
½   cup dry, white wine
2   tablespoons shallots, minced
½   cup seeded, chopped, fresh tomato (or drained, diced, canned tomatoes)
2   tablespoons heavy cream
1   tablespoon butter
1   teaspoon chopped, fresh tarragon (or 1 tablespoon of chopped, fresh basil)
2   tablespoons extra virgin olive oil

Preheat the oven to 400°F. Rinse the fish fillets, and allow them to rest on a paper towel to remove any excess moisture.

While the fish is drying, prepare the sauce. Bring the wine and shallots to a boil in a small saucepan. Boil it over medium heat until the wine is reduced to about 2 tablespoons. Add the tomato and continue to boil, mashing the tomato as it softens. Boil it until almost no liquid remains. Add the cream and tarragon, whisk gently, and bring it to a boil. Reduce the heat to low, and whisk in the butter until the butter is melted. Turn the heat off, and continue preparing the fish.

Squeeze a small amount of fresh lemon juice on both sides of the fish. Then lightly season both sides of the fish with salt, pepper, and paprika.

Heat about 2 tablespoons of olive oil in an oven-proof skillet, over medium heat (a nonstick pan works well, provided it is oven proof). Cook the oil until it starts to shimmer (but not smoke). Add the fish, searing each side to brown (1 to 1 ½ minutes per side). Then place the entire pan in the oven. Bake the fish 8 to 12 minutes, depending on the thickness of the fish.

Reheat the sauce on low heat. Spoon the sauce over the fish, and serve.

Nutrition Analysis: 6 carbs, 24 protein, 278 calories

Almost all fish, with the exception of farm-raised salmon, are considered lean. That is, their amount of saturated and total fat is very low. They are all high in Omega 3 fatty acids, which contribute to the health of our brains, hearts, joints, and many other areas of our bodies.

Fish-Taco Fish Plate

In this recipe, I eliminated the tortillas traditionally served with fish tacos. I added carbs that complement the fish but are more healthful and satisfying for the given carb counts.

4 servings

4	(4- to 5-ounce) fish fillets, skin removed
	Emeril's Essence (available on the spice aisle of the supermarket)
2	tablespoons flour
2	tablespoons extra virgin olive oil
¼	cup sour cream
1	chipotle pepper in adobo, chopped

Make the sauce first. In a small bowl, mix the chopped chipotle pepper into the sour cream. Test for heat, and add more to taste.

Rinse the fish fillets, and pat them dry with a paper towel. Sprinkle both sides of the fish with Emeril's Essence, and dredge them lightly in the flour.

Heat the olive oil in a large skillet, over medium heat. Cook the fish fillets 3 to 4 minutes per side until they flake easily when pierced with a fork. Serve these with the sauce.

Nutrition Analysis: 2 carbs, 24 protein, 230 calories (with sour cream sauce).
You can serve fish with Avocado Slaw, page 115: 8 carbs, 2 protein, 101 calories
- and -
Cuban-Style Black Beans, page 206: 22 carbs, 8 protein, 121 calories
- or -
Sautéed Corn and Squash, the Mexican version, page 190: 15 carbs, 4 protein, 178 calories

Mahi-Mahi in Raisin and Wine Sauce

2 servings

2	(4- to 5-ounce) mahi-mahi fillets, skin removed
	Salt and freshly ground, black pepper
¼	cup Panko bread crumbs
3	tablespoons extra virgin olive oil
1	tablespoon golden raisins
1 ½	tablespoons capers, rinsed
1	tablespoon pine nuts or chopped pistachios
2	tablespoons fresh lemon juice
2	tablespoons white wine
	Fresh parsley

Preheat the oven to 400°F. Lightly coat a baking sheet with nonstick, olive oil spray. Rinse the fish, and pat dry with a paper towel. Season the fish with salt and pepper. Coat both sides of the fish with Panko bread crumbs.

Heat the olive oil in large frying pan. Brown the fish on both sides. The bread crumbs will brown quickly, so cook the fish for less than 2 minutes per side. Place the fish on a baking sheet, and finish cooking it in the oven (about 10 minutes).

Meanwhile, remove all but 1 tablespoon of oil from the pan. Add the raisins, capers, and pine nuts (or pistachios), and stir it (in order to heat and brown the pine nuts). Add the wine and lemon juice to the pan, and stir well. Bring it to a boil, and reduce it slightly. Add freshly chopped parsley.

Place the fish on plates, and top it with sauce.

Nutrition Analysis: 14 carbs, 26 protein, 324 calories

All dried fruits, including raisins, have a high glycemic index. We have included this recipe to show you that you don't have to completely give up your favorite foods, even if they have a high glycemic index. You just have to eat them in moderation and with good protein. In a recipe like Mahi-Mahi in Raisin and Wine Sauce, you get to enjoy the raisin flavor without sitting down and eating an entire package of raisins.

Fish with White Wine and Garlic Sauce

This basic, sautéed fish recipe works well for most fish fillets, and it takes little time to prepare. Be sure to make your side dishes first, because the quick cooking time and hands-on method of this dish will require your attention. After you begin making the dish, you will not have time to prepare salads or vegetables.

2 servings; may be doubled

2	(5-ounce) fish fillets about ½-inch thick, skin removed
	Emeril's Original Essence
2	tablespoons of flour
1	tablespoon of extra virgin olive oil
½	clove of garlic, minced
¼	cup of dry, white wine
2	tablespoons of lemon juice
1	tablespoon of unsalted butter
1	teaspoon of capers, rinsed (optional)

Rinse the fish fillets, and pat them dry with a paper towel to remove any excess moisture. Sprinkle both sides of the fillets with Emeril's Essence. Lightly dredge the fish in the flour, just to dust the fillets, which creates a dry surface to allow browning (discard the remaining flour).

Heat 2 tablespoons of extra virgin olive oil in a large skillet, over medium-high heat. Place the fillets in the pan, and sauté them 3 to 4 minutes per side, depending on the thickness of the fish and the desired doneness. (The fish should feel firm and flake easily when pierced with a fork.) Remove the fish from the pan, and tent it with foil to keep it warm while you prepare the quick sauce.

Reduce the heat to medium-low, and add garlic to the pan. Stir it, and cook it for a few seconds until the garlic is fragrant but not browned. Add the dry white wine and lemon juice, stirring constantly to deglaze the pan (your aim is to release the brown bits on the surface of the pan). Add the butter and optional capers, and stir it until it is well blended. Transfer the fish to plates, and spoon sauce over the fillets. Serve it immediately.

Nutrition Analysis: 5 carbs, 24 protein, 325 calories

Emeril's Original Essence

Emeril's Original Essence is a nice seasoning blend for fish. It contains garlic, a touch of cayenne, oregano, and thyme, among other spices. You can buy Emeril Lagasse's signature seasoning at many supermarkets. You also can make it at home from his recipe, posted on the Emeril website.

Fish or Shrimp Cooked in Veracruz Sauce

This recipe from the Gulf Coast area of Veracruz, Mexico has become a classic dish. It is found in numerous cookbooks because it appeals to so many people. Today red snapper at the market often is highly expensive. As an alternative, substitute your favorite, mild-flavored fish or shrimp for the snapper. Halibut is a good alternative.

4 servings

Veracruz Sauce
2	tablespoons extra virgin olive oil
1	cup thinly sliced, white onion (1 medium onion)
3	cloves garlic, minced
4	cups diced, ripe tomatoes (Roma work well)
1	bay leaf
¼	teaspoon dried oregano
⅓	cup pimiento-stuffed green olives, sliced
1	tablespoon capers, rinsed and drained
1	tablespoon pickled jalapeno slices
4	(4- to 5-ounce) fish fillets, skin removed (or 1 pound of shrimp, peeled and deveined)
	Fresh lime
	Salt and freshly ground, black pepper

Heat 2 tablespoons of olive oil in a large skillet, over medium heat. Add the onions and garlic, and let these cook until the onions are soft but not brown (3 to 4 minutes). Add the tomatoes, bay leaf, olives, capers, and jalapenos. Simmer the sauce until it begins to thicken (8 to 10 minutes), stirring occasionally.

In the meantime, rinse and pat dry the fish fillets. Squeeze a small amount of fresh lime juice over the fish (or shrimp), and season the fillets with salt and freshly ground, black pepper.

When the sauce has thickened, add the fish fillets or shrimp to the pan, and spoon some of the sauce over the fish. Cook the fish until it is firm and flaky. (Or, if you are using shrimp, cook the shrimp until it is firm and pink.)

If the fish emits a lot of moisture, you will need to thicken the sauce again. To do this, first transfer the fish to a platter, and tent it with foil to keep it warm. Increase the heat on the sauce, and briskly simmer it to make it thicken.

Spoon the sauce over the fish, and serve it immediately.

Nutrition Analysis: 5 carbs, 24 protein, 325 calories

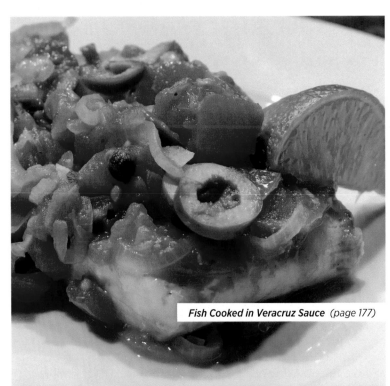

Fish Cooked in Veracruz Sauce (page 177)

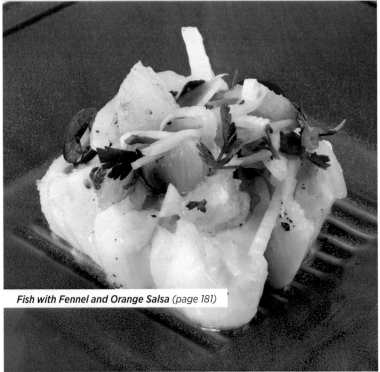

Fish with Fennel and Orange Salsa (page 181)

Spicy Baked Shrimp with Grits

You may be surprised to learn that you can eat grits on this program. But the key to success is to monitor your portion so that you don't eat too many carbohydrates with your meal. A side salad goes nicely with this dish.

2 servings; may be doubled

8 to 10 ounces of fresh shrimp, 20/25 count (cleaned and peeled, tails left on)

Marinade
- ¼ cup extra virgin olive oil
- 1 tablespoon fresh lemon juice
- ½ teaspoon salt
- ½ teaspoon sweet paprika
- ¼ teaspoon garlic powder
- ¼ teaspoon ground celery seed
- ¼ teaspoon dried oregano
- ¼ teaspoon cayenne
- ½ teaspoon minced, fresh garlic
- Freshly chopped parsley or thinly sliced green onions

Place the shrimp in a glass, oven-proof baking dish. Use a dish that is large enough to hold the shrimp in one layer. In a bowl, whisk the olive oil, lemon juice, salt, paprika, garlic powder, celery seed, oregano, cayenne, and fresh garlic. Pour this mixture over shrimp. Marinate the shrimp in the refrigerator for 20 to 30 minutes.

While shrimp is marinating, heat the oven to 400°F, and assemble the ingredients for the grits.

Grits
- ⅓ cup corn grits or polenta, such as Bob's Red Mill
- ⅓ cup water
- ⅔ cup whole milk
- ¼ cup grated Parmesan cheese

Bring the water and whole milk to a boil, and gradually add the grits. Reduce the heat. Place the shrimp in the oven, and bake it for 12 to 15 minutes while the grits simmer. Stir the grits often to prevent the food from sticking, and cook it for about 15 minutes. Add small quantities of additional water to the grits, if necessary.

Mix in the Parmesan cheese to the grits, and portion the grits into two bowls. Serve the shrimp and 1 tablespoon of the sauce from the baked shrimp over the grits, and garnish with freshly chopped parsley or thinly sliced green onions.

Nutrition Analysis: 25 carbs, 33 protein, 429 calories

Baked Salmon Teriyaki

This baked salmon with a mild marinade pairs nicely with the Lentil with Aromatics, on page 201.

4 servings

4   (4- to 5-ounce) wild-caught salmon fillets, about 1-inch thick, skin removed

Teriyaki Marinade
¼   cup chicken stock
¼   cup rice vinegar
2   tablespoons soy sauce or tamari
2   teaspoons honey
2   tablespoons fresh lime juice
2   teaspoons fresh ginger, minced (or ¼ teaspoon ground ginger)
1   clove garlic, minced
¼   teaspoon crushed red pepper flakes
2   tablespoons olive oil
     Salt and freshly ground, black pepper
     Fresh lemon

In a small bowl, whisk together all the marinade ingredients until they are well blended. Rinse the salmon, and pat it dry with paper towels. Place the fillets in a single layer in a glass or plastic container that is just large enough to hold the fillets. Pour the marinade over the fish, and turn the fish to coat well. Allow the food to marinate for 30 minutes or up to 1 hour (refrigerate it if you are marinating it for one hour).

Heat the oven to 400°F. Spray nonstick cooking spray on a rimmed baking sheet or large, glass, oven-proof dish.

Remove the salmon from marinade. Place the fish on the baking sheet. (You can then discard the marinade.) Season the salmon with salt and black pepper. Bake it for 10 to 12 minutes until the salmon flakes easily when pierced with a fork. Serve it with lemon wedges on the side.

Nutrition Analysis: 0 carbs, 24 protein, 186 calories

Fish with Fennel and Orange Salsa

This bright, citrusy salsa comes together quickly with a minimum of ingredients. Use a firm, white fish—not too delicate, so that it can stand up to the flavorful salsa. I like this salsa on cod and halibut. You will notice in the nutrition analysis how low-calorie this dish is—yet it is very satisfying. The salsa is to be prepared first.

2 servings; may be doubled

Salsa
- ⅓   cup very thinly sliced fennel bulb*
- 2   tablespoons thinly sliced, green onion (the green and white parts)
- 3   tablespoons chopped, fresh orange segments (about ¼ of an orange, peel and pith removed)
- 2   teaspoons fresh lemon juice
- 1   tablespoon thinly sliced Kalamata olives
- 1   tablespoon chopped, fresh parsley
- Cayenne pepper
- Salt and freshly ground, black pepper
- Fresh lemon wedges

The Remaining Ingredients
- 2   4- to 6-ounce fish fillets, skins removed
- 1   tablespoon extra virgin olive oil
- Salt and freshly ground, black pepper

> You can use fresh fennel sparingly, and it will still be very flavorful. One fennel bulb is usually big enough to use in several recipes throughout 1 week. You can roast it with other vegetables as a side dish, add it in small quantities to your fresh salads, or eat it as a snack with a few olives and a piece of Parmesan cheese. The fronds make a pretty garnish, and the stalks can be tossed into a pot of chicken stock.

Mix together the fennel, onion, orange, lemon juice, olives, and parsley. Sprinkle into the mixture a bit of cayenne (to taste) and salt and pepper. Set this mixture aside, unrefrigerated.

Rinse the fish, and pat dry it with a paper towel. Season the fish lightly with salt and pepper.

Heat the olive oil in a medium skillet, over medium-high heat. Add the fish, and cook it for 3 to 4 minutes per side, until the fish flakes easily when pierced with a fork.

Transfer the fish to a plate, and top it with the fennel and orange salsa. Serve the meal with a lemon wedge on the side.

Nutrition Analysis: (using halibut): 4 carbs, 30 protein, 189 calories

*If you need to know how to cut a fennel bulb, search for the topic on the internet. Online, you will find many good explanations and illustrations.

CHAPTER 15

Loading Up on Vegetables

Cooking vegetables is more about choosing a method and tossing vegetables together than it is about following recipes for every dish. The guidelines provided on roasting, grilling, sautéing, and fresh herbs will help you to create tasty vegetable sides according to what you have on hand.

By now you know why you need to spend more time in the produce section of the supermarket, and you know which vegetables are better for you. The produce section of today's supermarket is often the largest section of the store. This section is likely to have an amazing array of options presented any day of the week. Please eat local, organic, and seasonal produce as much as you can for the best nutrition and flavor.

Wellness 100 is about making better choices on an everyday basis.

- What is fresh now?
- What is affordable today?
- What else is in my refrigerator?
- What new vegetable would I like to try?
- What protein am I serving with these vegetables?

All of these questions might influence your grocery shopping. The point is, that a wide variety of fresh vegetables are readily available to you. You can easily eat more of these fresh foods—and eat fewer of the poor foods that have little to no nutritional value. Unfortunately, these poor foods have permeated the nation's diet.

You can load up on vegetables *and* be satisfied. After you rid your diet of extraneous carbohydrates in the form of white food, beverages, sugary dressings, and so on, the natural sugar in vegetables will find your palate. Perhaps it is best to get back to basics with vegetables: simple, fresh ingredients, prepared with little fuss.

Roasted Vegetables

Roasting vegetables concentrates their natural sugars and browns their surface, which equates to flavor. To prepare vegetables for roasting, you could quickly toss them in olive oil, salt, and pepper, and that would be enough. But for variety, you can add sweet paprika, garlic powder, and crushed red pepper. You can also nestle a sprig of rosemary into the vegetables while they bake.

Although some vegetables benefit from specific temperatures or methods, you can roast a variety of vegetables together by using the following directions, with very good results and little preparation.

- Heat your oven to 375°F. Or, if you are baking or roasting meat in your oven, you can use 350°F to 400°F (whatever you need for the meat) and adjust the cooking time for the vegetables accordingly.

- Cut the vegetables into uniform pieces so that they will cook evenly. Use a rimmed baking sheet that is large enough to spread your vegetables out into a single layer. (Or you can use 2 baking sheets.) Apply a thin coat of olive oil on the baking sheet. Toss the vegetables with additional olive oil (enough to coat the vegetables), and season them with salt and freshly ground, black pepper. Spread the vegetables out on the baking sheet in a single layer. Roast them for 15 minutes, and then stir them. Cook them for another 10 to 15 minutes or until the vegetables are tender.

Use any of the vegetables listed in Table 15.1 (alone, or in combination with two or three others). Good combinations are suggested in Table 15.2. Use Appendix B, Nutrition Analysis for Common Ingredients, to count carbs, protein, and calories.

Table 15.1
Preparing Vegetables for Roasting

asparagus	Choose asparagus that is about the thickness of a pencil. Trim the tough ends. Cut into 2-inch pieces if you are combining them with other vegetables. Leave them whole if you are roasting them alone.
broccoli	Leave a 1-inch stem on the broccoli floret. Cut the broccoli into uniform pieces about 1-inch thick.
Brussels sprouts	Trim the stems and peel off any limp or yellow outer leaves. Cut large sprouts in half. Any loose leaves turn crispy as they roast, and thus these are delicious!
carrots	Peel. Cut into pieces that are ½-inch thick × 2 inches long.
cauliflower	Separate the large florets. Then slice it about 1-inch thick, creating a flat surface for the cauliflower to make contact with the baking sheet.

cherry tomatoes	Add whole tomatoes to the baking sheet after the first 15 minutes of cooking.
eggplant	Peel or not, as you prefer. Slice it into ¼-inch rounds, or cut it into 1-inch cubes.
fennel bulb	Cut off the upper, green ribs and the root end close to the foot. Then cut lengthwise into ½-inch slices.
garlic cloves	Use as an aromatic. Peel two cloves, slice each in half, and add to the baking sheet (omit the garlic powder when using fresh garlic).
green beans	Cut into 2-inch pieces.
leeks (these have a mild onion flavor)	Cut off the dark-green, upper stalk. Leave a bit of pale-green stalk attached to the white bulbs. Trim off the hairy end of the bulb, leaving the bulb intact. Begin with the green end of the leek. Cut the leek in half lengthwise, stopping at about ½ inch from the end of the bulb. Immerse the leek in cold water. Swish the leek in the water, holding the bulb end. In this way, remove the sand and dirt that is settled between the layers. Cut off the bulb end, and you will have two long halves of the leek to roast.
onions or shallots	Cut an onion in half through the root end, and slice the onion ¼-inch thick or cut into wedges.
portobello mushrooms	Remove the stems. Use a spoon to scrape off the gills (or not—your choice). Slice into ½-inch strips or wedges.
potatoes	Once in a while, in very small quantities, treat yourself to roasted potatoes. If you roast them with other vegetables, then you won't eat too many. Cut potatoes into ½-inch rounds or into ½-inch wedges.
sweet peppers	Remove the seeds and veins. Slice into ½-inch strips or 1-inch pieces.
sweet potatoes	Peel. Cut into ¼-inch rounds or 1 ½-inch wedges.
white mushrooms	Remove the tough stems. Cut large mushrooms in half. Leave smaller mushrooms whole.
yellow squash	Trim the ends. Then cut in half, first lengthwise and then on the diagonal, into ½-inch pieces.
zucchini	Trim the ends. Cut in half lengthwise, and then on the diagonal, into ½-inch pieces.

Table 15.2
Favorite Vegetable Combinations

- Cauliflower, Brussels sprouts, sweet potatoes, and garlic
- Eggplant, peppers, and cherry tomatoes
- Carrots, cauliflower, green beans, and onions
- Mushrooms, zucchini, peppers, and onions
- Broccoli, cauliflower, and shallots
- Asparagus, alone, with only olive oil, salt, and pepper

Vegetable Sautés

Vegetable sautés are quick! They require little to no planning when using pantry and refrigerator staples such as olive oil, garlic, broth, soy sauce, nuts, herbs, and seasonings. You will read next about how to sauté, and Table 15.3 provides a list of preparation tips and flavor add-ons.

Basic Sauté Method

Heat 1 tablespoon of extra virgin olive oil in a large skillet, over medium heat. Add your prepared vegetables and minced garlic, if desired. Stir often. Season with salt and freshly ground, black pepper (or crushed red pepper). Add a splash of citrus or vinegar (wine, sherry, cider, and so forth) and serve.

Table 15.3
Preparing and Sautéing Vegetables

Vegetable and Preparation	Flavor Add-Ons
bok choy: slice (use leaves and stems)	• Use a splash of chicken broth to steam the bok choy. • minced garlic, soy sauce (small amount), crushed red pepper, mushrooms
baby bok choy: slice in half, lengthwise	• Use a splash of chicken broth to steam the bok choy. • soy sauce (small amount), crushed red pepper, mushrooms
kale: remove stems; slice leaves into ½-inch ribbons	• garlic or onions and a splash of chicken broth • lemon juice (a small amount) and pine nuts at the end • crushed red pepper or hot sauce
swiss chard: remove stems (save and add to soup); slice leaves into ½-inch ribbons	• garlic and a splash of chicken broth • pine nuts, golden raisins (just a few), red or white wine vinegar (small amount)
spinach: wash well; use 5 to 6 ounces of fresh spinach per serving	• generous garlic or shallots • a dab of butter or heavy cream
yellow squash: slice or chop	onions, pepper, zucchini; garnish with fresh herbs
zucchini: slice or chop	• lemon peel, thyme, feta cheese • eggplant, red pepper, onions
cherry tomatoes: whole or sliced in half	zucchini, corn, basil, thyme, balsamic vinegar, Parmesan

Table continued

mushrooms: slice	• Use butter and olive oil. • Add a few mushrooms to just about any other vegetables, to lend an earthy flavor. • Add a squeeze of lemon juice at the end.
eggplant: peel, and then slice ½-inch thick or cut into cubes	• Eggplant soaks up olive oil (add extra to the pan). • Add tomatoes, zucchini, onions, herbs; feta, or Parmesan cheese.
cauliflower florets: cut into uniform pieces	Add liquids, such as broth, or curry sauces.
onions, all types: sliced or coarsely chopped	Add to other vegetables as an aromatic.
broccoli florets: cut into uniform pieces	sun dried tomatoes, red bell pepper, soy sauce
green beans: cut into 2-inch pieces	garlic, onions, lemon, almonds or walnuts, vinegar or hot sauce
asparagus: trim ends and cut into 2-inch pieces	• garlic • lemon peel or lemon juice
brussels sprouts: trim ends and remove the outer leaves, then cut in half	• Cook, covered, with broth or water; then uncover and allow the liquid to reduce. • crushed red pepper
corn: fresh corn cut from the cob	• Use higher heat, initially, for corn. • bell peppers or poblano pepper and tomatoes
cabbage (napa, green, Savoy)	fresh ginger, carrots
sauerkraut (refrigerated, not canned)	onions, bell peppers

Green Beans with Red Onion and Walnuts

4 servings

1   tablespoon extra virgin olive oil
½   cup sliced, red onion
12   ounces (about 4 cups) fresh green beans, cut
        into 2-inch pieces
½   cup chicken broth (or vegetable broth)
⅛   cup (2 tablespoons) chopped walnuts
        Salt and freshly ground, black pepper

Nuts (almonds, walnuts, pine nuts, and pecans) are good accompaniments to green beans.

Heat the olive oil in large skillet, over medium heat. Add onion, and stir to coat. Cook the onion until it begins to soften (about 3 minutes).

Add the green beans and broth to the pan, and stir. Bring it to a simmer. Cover it, and reduce the heat. Simmer it gently for 10 minutes.

Remove the cover, and simmer it briskly until the broth is reduced to a few tablespoons (about 5 minutes), stirring occasionally.

The reduced broth may provide salt, so taste the beans first. Then, if needed, add salt and season with pepper. Add walnuts, and serve.

Nutrition Analysis: 10 carbs, 3 protein, 96 calories

Sautéed Corn and Squash

2 servings; may be doubled

1	medium ear fresh white or yellow corn (remove the corn from the cob)
1	cup grape tomatoes (or small, cherry tomatoes)
1	yellow squash, sliced ⅛-inch thick
	Salt and freshly ground, black pepper
1	teaspoon balsamic vinegar
1	tablespoon sliced, fresh basil (more to taste)
1	tablespoon shredded Parmesan cheese
1 ½	tablespoons extra virgin olive oil

Heat the olive oil in a skillet, over medium-high heat. Add the corn and squash, and stir them to coat them well. Sauté them for 3 to 4 minutes. Add the tomatoes, and stir well. Reduce the heat to medium. Cook it until the corn and squash are tender (about 5 more minutes), stirring occasionally. Season it with salt and freshly ground, black pepper. Add balsamic vinegar and fresh basil, and stir well. Top with Parmesan cheese, and serve.

Nutrition Analysis: 15 carbs, 4 protein, 168 calories

Variation for a Mexican-Style Sauté: Substitute cilantro for fresh basil. Substitute 2 teaspoons of fresh lime juice for balsamic vinegar. Add a dash of cumin.

The skin of any squash has higher amounts of antioxidants than the rest of the vegetable. If you are not buying organic, you may want to peel the skin to decrease your exposure to pesticides. If you buy organic squash, please eat the skin.

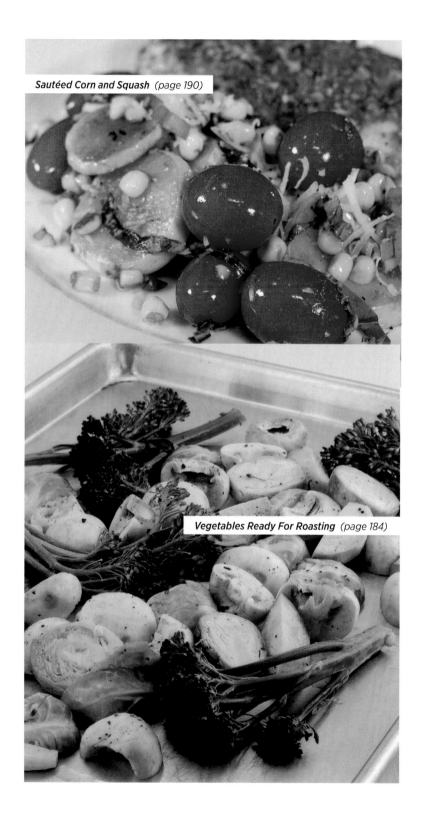

Sautéed Corn and Squash (page 190)

Vegetables Ready For Roasting (page 184)

Seared Baby Okra

Okra is best in the summer. At that time, use fresh, organic baby okra or small okra. Large okra pods can be tough, and so they are best suited to other cooking methods.

2 servings

1   tablespoon extra virgin olive oil
12   fresh baby okra (or more—as many as you will eat), rinsed and dried, left
        whole
     Salt
     Hot pepper sauce, such as Tabasco

Add the olive oil to a large, cast-iron skillet, and heat over medium heat until it is shimmering. Place okra in the pan, but do not overcrowd the pan. Allow the okra to sear on one side, and then turn or roll each piece of okra to sear on all sides. Cook for about 4 minutes total; do not overcook, or the okra will become slimy.

Remove it from the pan. Salt it lightly and serve. Season with hot sauce, if desired.

Nutrition Analysis: 5 carbs, 2 protein, 82 calories

We tend to think of okra as a southern food, particularly when okra is fried. It has its origins, however, in Egypt. It is very high in fiber, and thus it helps prevent colon cancer.

Grilled Vegetables

Take advantage of a heated grill! Cook vegetables to accompany your grilled meat. You can slice certain vegetables (such as eggplant, yellow squash, and zucchini) into large slices and place them directly on the grill. Or you can make kebabs. I use a grill basket when cooking vegetables on the grill; if you use a basket, you do not have to worry about losing your vegetables through the grill's grate.

Slice or chop your favorite vegetables into large pieces. Toss them with minced fresh garlic, olive oil, perhaps a splash of balsamic vinegar, salt, and pepper. Allow the vegetables to marinate while you heat (or cool) the grill to a medium setting. Place the vegetables into a grill basket on a medium-hot grill. Cook them, tossing once or twice to allow even cooking. Watch the heat; you don't want charred vegetables. Top them with fresh herbs, such as thyme or parsley, and serve them.

- asparagus
- red onions
- green onions
- bell peppers (red, green, or yellow)
- eggplant
- yellow squash
- zucchini
- cherry tomatoes
- Poblano peppers
- Portobello mushrooms
- white mushrooms
- corn—in the husk, soaked in salted water for 20 minutes before grilling

Grilled Vegetable Salad

Extra virgin olive oil
¼ teaspoon minced, fresh garlic
Chopped, fresh parsley
white Balsamic vinegar
Feta cheese

Prepare the vegetables* of your choice. Toss them with olive oil, salt, and freshly ground, black pepper. Grill them over medium heat. Remove the vegetables from the grill, and cool them. Chop the grilled vegetables into cubes, and mix them into prepared quinoa or a small portion of whole wheat pasta. Drizzle them with additional olive oil and white balsamic vinegar. Add fresh garlic, parsley, and feta cheese.

*For this recipe, use Appendix B, Nutrition Analysis for Common Ingredients, to count your carbs, protein, and calories.

Vegetables with Fresh Herbs

Fresh herbs, most of them applied at the end of cooking or as a garnish, can transform simple vegetables into savory, satisfying side dishes. For instance, bring out the best of steamed vegetables with a drizzle of olive oil and fresh herbs, instead of masking them with cheese sauce.

I understand that when you consider buying expensive, fresh herbs in those small packets at the grocery store to use in just one recipe, you may pause. But you can substitute fresh herbs for dry herbs in most recipes. Just use three times more fresh herbs than dry (1 teaspoon dry = 1 tablespoon fresh), and add them toward the end of the cooking process. (Sage and rosemary are an exception, because they benefit from a longer cooking time.)

I have a large herb garden in which I grow thyme, oregano, basil, tarragon, rosemary, dill, parsley, sage, chives, and mint. I use fresh herbs rather than dried herbs as often as I can. Some herbs can be grown successfully indoors, if you do not have a garden.

How to Use Fresh Herbs

If the herb has a woody stem (such as tarragon, thyme, oregano, basil, rosemary, and sage), then strip the herb from the stem and lightly chop the herb for use.

If the herb has tender stems (such as parsley, cilantro, and dill), then cut the bare stems from the base of the herb, but don't worry about picking all the leaves off the stems. Just chop the leaves and the tender stems together.

Fresh Herb Guide

- Parsley is a fresh herb that goes with just about anything. Buy flat-leaf (Italian) parsley rather than curly parsley, for better flavor. Sprinkle chopped parsley on any cooked vegetables, or add it to your fresh salads.

- Tarragon is one of my favorite fresh herbs. Its flavor resembles anise (liquorice), and it is delicious with a wide variety of vegetables. It perfectly complements green peas, and it is great with asparagus, cauliflower, broccoli, and sautéed mushrooms. Tarragon can be overpowering if you use too much, so only add a small amount at a time until you get the desired taste.

- Thyme pairs well with so many vegetables: green beans, broccoli, mushrooms, red and green bell peppers, onions, tomatoes, eggplant, zucchini, and Brussels sprouts.

- Basil is a mildly spicy herb, delightful with eggplant, tomatoes, corn, and yellow squash. Basil pairs well with raw vegetables, and it is delicious when sprinkled on fresh salads. Basil and oregano work well together.

- Oregano is essential to Greek salads, and it is great on cooked tomatoes, peppers, eggplant, mushrooms, zucchini, and bell peppers.

- Rosemary should be added to food while the food is cooking. I like to add a sprig or two of rosemary to a baking sheet of vegetables while they are roasting (especially if I add a small potato to the mix). Discard the stem before serving.

- Fresh dill is pungent. Use it sparingly at first, and then add more to taste. I love fresh dill on tomatoes and mixed with fresh salad greens.

- Fresh sage is not to be used raw; it needs to be cooked with food, as it is in the cannellini bean recipe on page 203. It pairs well with onions, winter squash, and root vegetables.

- Chives typically have a mild onion or garlic flavor. Use them as a garnish to impart this flavor on steamed vegetables or in a fresh salad.

- Cilantro (coriander) is in the parsley family, but it has its own distinct flavor. Ground coriander is made from the seeds, and it is not a substitute for fresh cilantro. Cilantro complements tomatoes, peppers, squash, sweet potatoes, eggplant, avocados, salads, and grilled vegetables. Be sure to wash cilantro well to remove the sand and dirt from its leaves and stems.

- Fresh mint is uplifting and cooling. I use fresh mint in cold salads and in beverages more than I do on cooked vegetables. That being said, mint is great with peas or tossed into a warm salad of grilled summer vegetables and feta cheese.

Simply Perfect Peas

Peas have a high carbohydrate count when compared to many other vegetables, due to their natural sugar content. However, they also contain protein and fiber, and they have a low glycemic index. English peas (the small round green peas) are the one vegetable that I routinely buy frozen. Keep them in your freezer to quickly include them as a hot vegetable side dish, to use in soup, or to include them in your quinoa salads.

4 servings

2	cups frozen peas
	Water
½	tablespoon unsalted butter, cut into pieces
1	teaspoon fresh tarragon, chopped (or ¼ teaspoon dried tarragon)
	Salt and freshly ground, black pepper

Cook the frozen peas in water on the stovetop, according to the product directions. Drain.

Add the butter and tarragon, and season the peas with salt and pepper.

Nutrition Analysis: 9 carbs, 4 protein, 64 calories

Stewed Vegetables (Ratatouille)

6 servings; may be doubled

12	ounces eggplant, peeled and cut into 1-inch cubes (about 4 cups total)
12	ounces zucchini (about 2 medium zucchini), washed and cut into 1-inch cubes
1 ½	cups sliced onion
1	red bell pepper, cut into 1-inch pieces
1	green bell pepper, cut into 1-inch pieces
2	cloves garlic, minced
1 ½	cups tomatoes, chopped into 1-inch pieces
2	teaspoons fresh thyme, or ½ teaspoon dried thyme
3	tablespoons minced, fresh parsley
	Salt and freshly ground, black pepper
3	tablespoons extra virgin olive oil

Heat the olive oil in a large skillet over medium-high heat, and add the eggplant and zucchini. Cook them for 8 to 10 minutes, and stir infrequently. Remove the vegetables from the pan, and add the onions and peppers, cooking them until soft (about 8 minutes). Add garlic and tomatoes, and season them with salt and pepper. Add thyme, and reduce the heat to low. Cook it until the tomatoes release their juice and begin to evaporate (about 5 minutes). Add eggplant and zucchini back to the pan, and cook it another 10 minutes. Mix in the fresh parsley, and serve.

Baked Egg with Ratatouille: If you have ratatouille leftovers, reheat a single serving in an 8-inch skillet, over medium heat. When it is heated through and bubbling, make a well in the center, and break an egg into the well. Cover it, and reduce the heat to medium low. Cook for about 5 minutes until the egg is set.

Nutrition Analysis: 14 carbs, 3 protein, 119 calories

Broccoli, Cauliflower, and Brussels Sprouts Au Gratin

A creamy au gratin is a nice comfort food alongside a roast pork or chicken.

6 to 8 servings

3   cups broccoli florets
3   cups cauliflower florets
8   ounces (about 2 cups) Brussels sprouts, the outer
        leaves removed, stems removed, and sliced
        ¼-inch thick
1   tablespoon butter, cut into pieces
½   cup heavy cream
½   cup chicken broth
½   teaspoon Dijon-style mustard
1   tablespoon fresh lemon juice
¼   teaspoon dried tarragon (or basil)
½   cup grated Parmesan cheese
     Freshly ground, black pepper
2   slices Ezekiel bread or whole wheat bread (for bread crumbs)
1   tablespoon extra virgin olive oil

> To save preparation time for your meals, pair flavorful, more complex vegetable dishes like this one with simply prepared meats. Likewise, serve more flavorful meat dishes with simply prepared vegetables.

Heat oven to 350°F. Lightly coat a shallow 1 ½-quart oven-proof casserole dish (or a 2-inch deep glass pie plate) with a drizzle of extra virgin olive oil.

Parboil the Vegetables. Bring 4 quarts of water to a boil in a large saucepan, over high heat. Add 2 teaspoons of salt. Add the broccoli, cauliflower, and Brussels sprouts. Return it to a boil, and cook for 2 more minutes. Drain the vegetables, add butter, and stir to coat.

Make Bread Crumbs. Tear the bread into pieces, and pulse it in the bowl of a food processor or mini food processor to make fresh bread crumbs. Mix the bread crumbs with 1 tablespoon of extra virgin olive oil.

Mix the cream, broth, mustard, lemon juice, tarragon, cheese, and pepper in a small bowl. Pour the cream mixture over the vegetables, and mix well. Put it in the prepared casserole dish.

Spread the bread crumbs evenly over the vegetables. Cover it with foil and bake for 25 minutes. Remove the foil, and bake it for another 20 minutes (until the broccoli and cauliflower are very tender when pierced with a fork).

Nutrition Analysis: 12 carbs, 10 protein, 193 calories

CHAPTER 16

Briefly, Beans and Grains

We use beans in many recipes in this book, but always in a portion-controlled manner due to the carbohydrate content. Beans have many virtues: they have a low glycemic index, they are a low-fat source of protein, and they are a good source of fiber. So you can feel good about eating beans often. Be sure to think of beans as a carbohydrate first, and then you will effectively add them to your plate either as a side dish or in soups, stews, and salads.

We always suggest using fresh or raw foods over processed food. But beans require either presoaking or a long cooking time (or both). Thus it is better to incorporate these legumes into your diet even if they are canned. There is not much nutritional difference between canned beans or boiled beans; but be aware that canned beans have a higher glycemic index than boiled beans. Always drain and rinse canned beans before using them in any recipe. Lentils cook more quickly than other types of dried beans (about 25 minutes), because they are flat and have thin seed coats.

Table 16.1 shows a nutritional analysis for commonly used beans, in ½-cup boiled or canned portions. Add the appropriate amount to your soups and stews based upon the number of servings you are making.

Table 16.1
Commonly Used Beans in ½-Cup Portions

Cooked Bean	Carbs	Protein	Calories
Black beans, ½ cup	21	8	114
Black-eyed peas, ½ cup	17	7	100
Cannellini beans, ½ cup	17	6	100
Chickpeas (Garbanzo beans), ½ cup*	27	6	143
Kidney beans, ½ cup	19	7	108
Lentils, ½ cup	20	9	115
Navy beans, ½ cup	20	7	110
Pinto beans, ½ cup	22	8	123

*Dried chickpeas, boiled, contain 22 carbs, 7 protein, and 134 calories per ½-cup serving as compared to the canned beans shown in Table 16.1.

Pasta

A single serving of pasta, according to various nutritional labels, contains about 42 grams of carbohydrates. It is crucial to recognize that pasta must be strictly controlled when it comes to portions. Even quinoa has too many carbohydrates for the Wellness program, if you eat a suggested serving according to the package. Please be aware of your carbohydrate portions; cook about one-half serving per person, instead of the suggested serving size.

Green Lentils with Aromatics

Lentils are high in protein and soluble fiber. They cook about 3 times faster than most other types of dried beans, and they do not require presoaking, which makes them a great pantry item to have on hand.

6 servings; the serving size is ½ cup

1	tablespoon unsalted butter
1	teaspoon extra virgin olive oil
¼	cup finely chopped carrot
¼	cup finely chopped onion
¼	cup finely chopped celery
2	cloves garlic, minced
1	cup green lentils, rinsed
2	cups chicken broth
1	bay leaf
⅛	teaspoon ground cloves
2	teaspoons sherry vinegar
	Salt and freshly ground, black pepper

If you want to seek out other recipes with lentils, try searching for dal. Dal is an Indian dish that uses red lentils and spices such as curry, garam masala, turmeric, and ginger.

Heat the butter and olive oil in a 2-quart saucepan, over medium heat. Add the carrot, onion, celery, and garlic. Cook it for 5 minutes, stirring often.

Add the lentils, broth, bay leaf, and ground cloves. Bring it to a boil, cover it with the lid offset, and reduce the heat to allow a low simmer. Cook it for 25 to 30 minutes, or until the lentils are tender.

Add sherry vinegar, and season with salt and pepper to taste. Stir, and cook for 2 more minutes to allow the vinegar to permeate the dish.

Nutrition Analysis: 21 carbs, 9 protein, 146 calories

Chicken and Snap Pea Quinoa Salad

Quinoa is high in protein and contains all 9 essential amino acids as well as good carbohydrates. Prepare organic quinoa according to directions on the package, then add your favorite vegetables and small portions of meat to make a healthy lunch salad. Quinoa is nutty, but not particularly flavorful in and of itself. This finished dish takes on the flavors that you add, such as lemon and parsley. (Or, for example, pork and cumin go well together.)

2 servings

⅓	cup uncooked quinoa
½	cup water
4 to 6	ounces cooked chicken (or turkey), cut into bite size pieces
2	tablespoons extra virgin olive oil
2	tablespoons fresh lemon juice
1	cup sugar snap peas, strings removed if necessary, cut into ½-inch pieces
2	carrots, peeled and thinly sliced
½	clove garlic, minced
2	green onions, thinly sliced
¼	cup chopped, fresh parsley
	Salt and freshly ground, black pepper

Wash the quinoa in cold water and drain. Bring ½ cup water to a boil. Add the washed quinoa. Cover the pan, reduce the heat to low, and simmer the quinoa for 12 minutes. Remove it from heat, and let it rest for 5 minutes. Transfer the quinoa to a large bowl and allow it to cool.

To the quinoa, then add chicken (or turkey), olive oil, and lemon juice. Add the remaining ingredients, and mix it well. Eat the salad immediately, or refrigerate it (it will keep up to 24 hours).

Nutrition Analysis: 30 carbs, 24 protein, 371 calories

Cannellini with Sage and Garlic

6 servings (may be halved)

3	cups cooked cannellini beans, or 2 (15-ounce) cans, rinsed and drained
1	cup chicken broth or vegetable broth
1	bay leaf
¼	cup thinly sliced onion
2	cloves garlic, minced
1	tablespoon fresh sage, thinly sliced
3	tablespoons extra virgin olive oil, divided
	Salt and freshly ground, black pepper

Add the cannellini beans to a medium saucepan. Add broth and bay leaf, and bring it to a boil. Reduce the heat, and simmer it gently for about 20 minutes. Use a ladle or spoon to remove and set aside about ½ cup of broth from the beans. Drain the beans.

Heat 1 tablespoon of the olive oil in a large, nonstick skillet, over medium heat. Add the onion, and sauté until soft (about 5 minutes). Add the garlic and sage, and cook briefly (about 1 minute), being careful not to burn the garlic. Add the beans, the remaining 2 tablespoons of olive oil, and the reserved broth. Mix it well, and bring it to a simmer. The beans should be moist, but not soupy. If there is too much liquid in the pan, simmer it until most of the liquid is absorbed. Season it with salt and black pepper, and serve.

Nutrition Analysis: a serving size of ½ cup has 18 carbs, 6 protein, 167 calories

> **Sage** is a member of the mint family. It works as an anti-inflammatory, and as such sage can help with arthritis and asthma (as well as fight against atherosclerosis, which leads to heart disease).

Pork and Roasted Vegetable Quinoa

2 servings

⅓   cup uncooked quinoa
½   cup water
4-6 ounces cooked pork (loin, chops, or tenderloin), cut into bite size pieces
2   tablespoons extra virgin olive oil
3   tablespoons fresh lemon juice
½   clove garlic, minced
⅛   teaspoon ground cumin
1   cup roasted vegetables (use extra roasted vegetables from last night's
       dinner—see the recipe on page 184)
¼   cup fresh parsley, chopped
2   tablespoons feta cheese

Wash the quinoa in cold water, and drain it. Bring ½ cup of water to a boil. Add the washed quinoa. Cover it. Reduce the heat to low, and simmer it for 12 minutes. Remove it from the heat, and let it rest for 5 minutes. Transfer the quinoa to a large bowl, and allow it to cool.

To the quinoa, add the pork, olive oil, lemon juice, garlic, cumin, chopped vegetables, and parsley, and mix it well. Top it with feta cheese. Eat it immediately; or, you can refrigerate it and keep it up to 24 hours.

Nutrition Analysis: 23 carbs, 23 protein, 388 calories

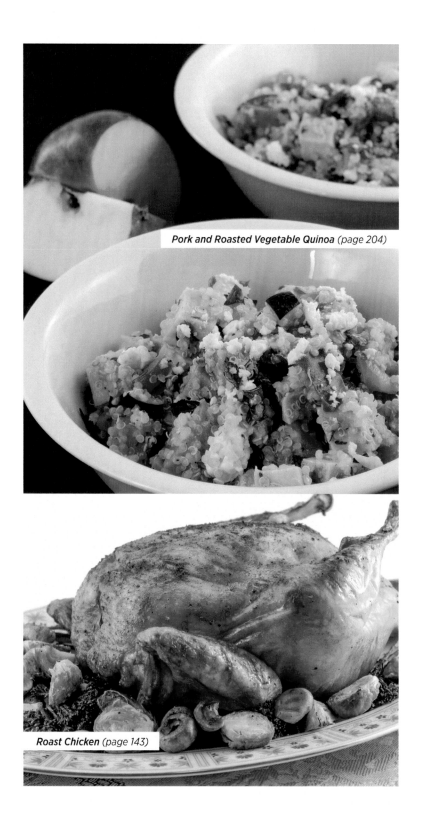

Pork and Roasted Vegetable Quinoa (page 204)

Roast Chicken (page 143)

Cuban-style Black Beans

6 servings (may be halved)

3	cups cooked black beans, or 2 (15-ounce) cans, drained and rinsed
1	cup chicken broth
⅓	cup finely chopped, white onion, more for garnish
1	clove garlic, minced (or ¼ teaspoon of garlic powder)
¼	teaspoon cumin
1	small jalapeno
1	teaspoon red-wine vinegar
	Salt

Mix the beans, broth, onion, garlic, and cumin in a medium-size saucepan. Pierce the jalapeno in a few places with the tip of a knife, and add it to the pot. Bring the beans to a simmer over medium heat. Reduce the heat, and cook it partially covered for 15 to 20 minutes (until the beans absorb much of the broth). Remove the jalapeno from the beans. Add the red-wine vinegar, and season it with salt.

Nutrition Analysis: 22 carbs, 8 protein, 120 calories

Broccoli and Sun-dried Tomato Quinoa

This recipe does not contain enough protein to make it a complete meal. You can serve it as a side dish to grilled meat. Or you can add a few ounces of cooked beef or chicken to make a great lunch dish.

2 servings

⅓	cup uncooked quinoa
½	cup water
1	recipe for Marinated Broccoli Salad, page 116
⅛	cup sun-dried tomatoes, chopped
	Extra virgin olive oil
	Fresh lemon juice or white-wine vinegar

Wash the quinoa in cold water, and drain it. Bring ½-cup of water to a boil. Add the washed quinoa. Cover it, reduce the heat to low, and simmer it for 12 minutes. Remove it from the heat, and let it rest for 5 minutes. Cool it completely.

Add the marinated broccoli and the sun-dried tomatoes to the cooled quinoa. Mix it well, and then taste it. Add more olive oil and lemon juice (or white-wine vinegar) to taste.

Nutrition Analysis: 26 carbs, 7 protein, 276 calories (not including added chicken or beef)

CHAPTER 17

Smart Snacks and Appetizers

Snacking has become an all-day affair for many people, especially for those who eat too many carbohydrates and too little protein in meals (which leads to wanting more carbs). A snack is meant to bridge the gap between meals and not be thought of as a meal in itself.

You can have two snacks per day if you would like; but you don't have to, if you are not hungry. Snacks should be about 100 calories and include no more than 5 to 8 grams of carbs with good fat and protein.

The appetizer recipes in this section will help you to make good choices about what to take to parties or what to use when you are entertaining.

- Almonds (15 almonds)
- Other nuts and seeds such as peanuts, walnuts, pistachios, pumpkin seeds, and sunflower seeds (about ⅛ cup of any one of these)
- 2 tablespoons hummus, drizzled with a bit of olive oil and cayenne, with as much celery as you want
- 1 deviled egg, with celery and carrot sticks
- 3 tablespoons Spicy Black Bean Dip (page 212), with as much celery and red bell pepper as you want
- Cheddar cheese (a 1-inch cube), or 1 piece of string cheese and 1 medium dill pickle
- 2 tablespoons Tart Lemon Feta Dip (page 211), with fresh vegetables such as celery, cucumber, and cherry tomatoes
- Quick artichoke dip: 1 whole artichoke heart (from a can of artichoke hearts), chopped, mixed with 2 tablespoons of cream cheese and hot pepper sauce to taste, served with celery or red bell pepper
- Fruit, with ¼-cup cottage cheese: fresh blueberries (¼ cup) or ½ of a tangerine
- Cherry tomatoes (up to ½ cup) and cottage cheese (¼ cup)
- Quick pesto dip: 1 tablespoon pesto mixed into cream cheese, served with celery and red bell pepper
- Quick fruit dip: 1 tablespoon cream cheese mixed with a little cinnamon or nutmeg, served with ⅓ of a medium apple or pear
- 2 teaspoons peanut butter, with fruit or celery

- 2 tablespoons tuna salad, with vegetable sticks
- 2 thin slices lean deli ham or turkey, rolled with lettuce and a "shmear" of cream cheese

Tart Lemon Feta Dip

Use just about any fresh vegetables (sugar snap peas, celery, bell peppers, cucumber, cauliflower, and so forth) with this tangy, salty dip. After you've made the basic recipe, add ingredients you like (such as sun-dried tomatoes, roasted red peppers, sliced pepperoncini, or fresh basil). Be sure to use a food processor to make this dip. I tried to whisk it, mash it, and whip it by hand, but still I could not achieve a smooth consistency.

Serving size: 2 tablespoons

1	(6-ounce) container crumbled feta cheese
4	tablespoons extra virgin olive oil
2	tablespoons fresh lemon juice
¼	teaspoon freshly ground, black pepper (or more to taste)
2	tablespoons chopped, fresh parsley

Place the feta cheese into a food processor. (It will fit in a mini food processor/chopper.) Add olive oil and fresh lemon juice, and pulse it until it is smooth. Add black pepper, and pulse it to mix.

Transfer the dip to a small bowl, and add fresh parsley and other optional ingredients (such as chopped, fresh basil, roasted red pepper, or sun-dried tomatoes).

Nutrition Analysis: 1 carb, 4 protein, 94 calories

Spicy Black Bean Dip

This dip is great to serve to guests, or to take to a party. You can offer fresh vegetables such as red bell pepper, celery, and carrots for dipping (as a healthy alternative to tortilla chips).

Makes about 3 cups (16 servings)

1	tablespoon extra virgin olive oil
⅓	cup finely chopped carrot
⅓	cup finely chopped celery
⅓	cup finely chopped onion
⅓	cup finely chopped, red bell pepper
1	clove garlic, minced
3	cups cooked black beans (or two 15-ounce cans), rinsed and drained
	Chicken or vegetable broth
1	chipotle pepper in adobo, chopped
	Salt
1	cup feta cheese, crumbled
	Fresh salsa
	Chopped avocado (optional)

In a medium saucepan, heat the olive oil over medium heat. Add the carrot, celery, onion, red bell pepper, and garlic, and stir it. Cook it until the vegetables start to soften (about 5 minutes), stirring often. Add beans, and mix. Add just enough broth to barely cover the mixture. Add chipotle pepper, and stir.

Bring it to a simmer. Lower the heat, and cook it for 15 minutes to allow the beans to absorb the broth. Stir it occasionally. Remove it from the heat when the mixture is almost dry (be careful not to scorch the beans.)

Cool it slightly. Use an immersion blender to puree or transfer the beans to a food processor, and then puree it until it is smooth, being careful not to splash any hot liquids on yourself.

Spoon the mixture into a shallow glass dish (such as a pie plate). Top it with crumbled feta, and then top it with fresh salsa and avocado. Serve it at room temperature. Or you can make it ahead and warm the dip (topped with feta cheese) in a preheated 350°F oven for about 25 minutes (until it is warmed through). Add salsa, and serve.

Nutrition Analysis (3 tablespoons per serving): 9 carbs, 4 protein, 78 calories (not including avocado)

Deviled Eggs

Deviled (or stuffed) eggs make a great protein addition to appetizer platters. You can plan on one-half to one whole egg per person. Add deviled eggs to your lunch salads, or use them as an afternoon snack. Turn them into egg salad, and make a breakfast sandwich to go.

Serving size (as a snack): 1 deviled egg (½ of an egg)

The Eggs

Use 4 large eggs. Start each recipe with 4 hard-boiled eggs, peeled and sliced in half lengthwise. Remove the egg yolks from each half, and place these in a small bowl. Mash the yolks with a fork, add the extra ingredients, and mix it well. Mound a filling into each cooked egg white, and sprinkle with paprika or add a garnish of chopped, fresh parsley to any of these recipes. Refrigerate the eggs to keep them for a day; these taste best served at room temperature.

Sun-dried Tomatoes
2	tablespoons extra virgin olive oil
¼	cup sun-dried tomatoes packed in oil, drained and chopped
¼	teaspoon red-wine vinegar or white-wine vinegar
¼	teaspoon dried marjoram
	Salt and freshly ground, black pepper

Nutrition Analysis: 0 carbs, 3 protein, 71 calories

Dijon and Pepper Sauce
1	tablespoon mayonnaise
1	teaspoon Dijon-style mustard
	A few drops of hot pepper sauce
	Salt and freshly ground, black pepper

Nutrition Analysis: 0 carbs, 3 protein, 52 calories

Roasted Red Peppers and Lemon
2	tablespoons extra virgin olive oil
1 ½	tablespoons chopped, roasted red pepper
1	teaspoon fresh lemon juice
¼	teaspoon minced garlic
	Salt and freshly ground, black pepper

Nutrition Analysis: 0 carbs, 3 protein, 71 calories

Lemon and Feta

Add 1 to 2 tablespoons Tart Lemon Feta Dip (page 211) to the egg yolks, and stir it until well blended.

Nutrition Analysis: 0 carbs, 4 protein, 52 calories

Marinated Olives and Pepperoncini

Pepper and garlic turn ordinary olives into a treat. Serve these as part of an appetizer platter with sliced, fresh fennel bulb and small cubes of cheese. That will give you a nice nibble! You have the option in this recipe of refrigerating it for a few hours or overnight.

10 servings

1	cup pimiento-stuffed green olives, drained (use cracked olives if you prefer)
½	cup whole pepperoncini, drained
3	tablespoons extra virgin olive oil
1	tablespoon red-wine vinegar
¾	teaspoon dried oregano
½	teaspoon minced garlic
¼	teaspoon crushed red pepper
	High-quality hard cheese, such as Parmesan, aged Cheddar, Asiago, or Manchego

Pierce the tips of the pepperoncini to release the juice. In a medium bowl, whisk the olive oil, red-wine vinegar, oregano, garlic, and crushed red pepper. Add the olives and pepperoncini. Stir it to coat. Transfer it to a storage container with a lid. Refrigerate it, stirring occasionally, for several hours or overnight. Bring the olives to room temperature, and serve them.

Nutrition Analysis: (with 5 olives) 1 carb, 0 protein, 43 calories

Manchego is a Spanish cheese made from sheep's milk. It is easy to find now in most grocery stores. It is a firm cheese, with an off-white to yellow color. It has a wonderful flavor and makes a great appetizer.

Bayou Baby Bellos

This recipe is a variation of an oyster recipe given to me by good friends from southern Louisiana ("bayou country"). Mushrooms soak up the savory broth. This recipe may be doubled. For a small gathering, serve these as part of a platter with other nibbles, such as small bites of cheese and olives.

6 servings

8	ounces baby portobello mushrooms, cleaned, the stems removed
2	tablespoons butter
½	cup chicken broth
2	tablespoons Vermouth or white wine
2	teaspoons Worcestershire sauce
1	teaspoon garlic powder
½	teaspoon celery seeds (whole or ground)
½	teaspoon hot pepper sauce (such as Tabasco)
2	teaspoons Creole seasoning, such as Tony Chachere's (or ¼ teaspoon cayenne)

If the mushrooms are the same size, do not slice them; otherwise, cut the large portobello mushrooms in half. (Mushrooms should be similarly sized for even cooking).

Melt the butter over medium heat in a medium, nonstick skillet. Add the broth, Vermouth, Worcestershire sauce, garlic powder, celery seeds, pepper sauce, and Creole seasoning. Then whisk. Add mushrooms, and simmer briskly until almost all of the liquid is gone (20 to 30 minutes). Stir occasionally.

Serve it warm or at room temperature.

Nutrition Analysis: 3 carbs, 1 protein, 51 calories

Boiled Shrimp with Roasted Red Pepper Sauce

Shrimp cocktail is a nice addition at any dinner or get together, but cocktail sauce does not fit the program. The reason is because just 1 serving of prepared cocktail sauce has anywhere from 6 to 16 grams of carbs, mostly from high-fructose corn syrup!

In this recipe, you will be making a red pepper sauce before you start to cook the shrimp. Cook the shrimp in their shells, and when these are completely cooled, peel the shrimp (leaving the tails on) or allow guests to "peel and eat." Serve with lemon wedges and the pepper sauce.

8 appetizer servings (or 4 main-course servings)

Make the sauce before you boil the shrimp (see the following).

Roasted Red Pepper Sauce
Makes ¾ cup
8 servings

1	green onion, trimmed, chopped
3	tablespoons chopped celery
⅓	cup chopped, roasted red peppers (bottled are fine)
1	teaspoon Dijon-style mustard
1	clove garlic, minced
1 ½	tablespoons of fresh lemon juice
½	teaspoon of Worcestershire sauce
2	tablespoons extra virgin olive oil
2	tablespoons mayonnaise
	Dash cayenne
	Salt to taste

Place the onion and celery in the bowl of a food processor, and pulse to mince. Transfer the mixture into a small bowl, and set this bowl aside. Add the red pepper, mustard, garlic, lemon juice, and Worcestershire to the processor, and puree it until smooth. Add the olive oil, and process it until well blended. Add the mayonnaise, cayenne, and salt, and pulse to blend.

Transfer the red pepper sauce to the bowl with the onion and celery, and mix it well. Taste it, and add more cayenne if desired. Chill the sauce while you prepare the shrimp.

Boiled Shrimp

    1 to 2 pounds raw, wild-caught shrimp, 16/20 count (no smaller than 21/25
            count)

2   lemons, quartered
2   limes, quartered
⅛   teaspoon ground oregano (or use ½ teaspoon dried oregano, crushed
        between your fingers)
2   bay leaves
¼   teaspoon of Tabasco
      Fresh lemon wedges for serving

Fill a large stock pot with 3 quarts of water. Squeeze the lemon and lime quarters into water, and toss the rinds into the water. Add oregano, bay leaves, and Tabasco to the water. Bring it to a boil over high heat.

While the water comes to a boil, fill a large bowl ¾ full with ice water.

Add shrimp to the boiling water. After the water comes back to a boil, cook the shrimp for 3 minutes. (The shrimp will turn pink.) Remove it from the heat. Drain the shrimp, rinse them with cold water, and toss them into the ice water to stop the cooking process. Drain the shrimp after 5 minutes, and refrigerate it. Chill it for 1 hour before serving. Keep any excess shrimp refrigerated for use within 24 hours.

Nutrition Analysis:
Appetizer: 1 carb, 12 protein, 128 calories
Main course: 2 carbs, 24 protein, 227 calories
Shrimp only (4 ounces; no sauce): 0 carbs, 24 protein, 112 calories

> **You can also make the boiled shrimp** without the sauce and serve it as a main course (with 3 to 4 ounces of shrimp per person) atop a Greek salad, for a light summer dinner.

Conclusion

The most natural and lasting way to achieve a weight-loss goal and improve your overall health is to eat a varied diet full of fresh, unprocessed foods. Over the long term, no shots, no pills, and no fad diets can do it better or safer.

We know how easy it is to be confused by food packaging and marketing gimmicks that bombard us as we walk through the supermarket. The advice "everything in moderation" has lost its meaning in today's world of fast food, packaged meals, low-fat, no-fat, and zero-calorie offerings. The false promises on food packaging can make your head spin. These claims have, in fact, created generations of people who don't know what they should eat to lose weight and feel good.

That is why we want to help you cut through the clutter and learn how to eat properly for the rest of your life. Let *Wellness 100: 100 Carbs/100 Recipes* guide you through the science of nutrition to a fresher, tastier, and healthier way of eating on an everyday basis. Be sure to visit the website companion to this book, http://wellness100.us .

Make it a priority to eat a proper breakfast with protein, every day. Learn to eat vegetables and whole grains with appropriate portions of lean meat and good fat (such as olive oil). Give up the empty calories and the expanding waist line. If you do, you will discover that you will not have to count calories. You do not have to feel as if you are on a perpetual diet. Rather, you can eat home-cooked food, with healthy ingredients that suit your tastes and your needs. We hope that you enjoy the straightforward recipes in this book. You can get back to basics and eat flavorful, healthful food that is also delicious and satisfying.

Appendix A

Wellness 100 Bread Options

Note that these products vary from brand to brand. So read the label and nutritional information to choose wisely when shopping for bread options.

Product	Carbs	Protein	Calories
Ezekiel bread, 1 slice	15	4	80
whole wheat bread, 1 slice	13	4	77
whole wheat pita, small (4 inch)	15	3	74
whole wheat pita, ½ large (6 ½ inch)	18	3	85
whole wheat English muffin	24	6	120
corn tortilla (1)	11	0	52
whole wheat wrap (1)	16	2	120
whole wheat sandwich, thin slice (1 whole)	21	5	100

Ezekiel bread is made from sprouted whole grains and beans rather than flour. It is high in fiber and has a low glycemic index.

Appendix B

Nutrition Analysis for Common Ingredients

(See Appendix A, "Wellness 100 Bread Options," for bread data.)

Ingredient and Quantity	Carbs*	Protein*	Calories*
Condiments			
bread crumbs, Panko, ¼ cup	15	2	71
bread crumbs, plain or seasoned, ¼ cup	19	4	107
anchovies, packed in oil, 2	0	2	16
balsamic vinegar, 1 tablespoon	5	0	20
butter, 1 tablespoon	0	0	102
capers, 1 tablespoon	0	0	2
chicken broth, Swanson organic, 1 cup	1	1	15
dijon mustard, 1 teaspoon	0	0	5
flour, white, all purpose, 1 tablespoon	6	1	29
honey, 1 tablespoon	17	1	64
honey, 1 teaspoon	6	0	21
mayonnaise, Hellmann's, 1 tablespoon	0	0	90
olives, green, cracked (0.5 oz)	2	0	35
olives, green, with pimiento (5)	1	0	25
olives, Kalamata, pitted 3 to 4, average	1	0	32
olives, Kalamata, pitted, ¼ cup	3	0	100
red-wine vinegar, 2 tablespoons	1	0	5
soy sauce, ¼ cup	1	13	39
soy sauce, 1 tablespoon	0	2	10
sugar, granulated, 1 teaspoon	4	0	16
sugar, granulated, white, 1 tablespoon	12	0	46
sugar, granulated, white, 1 teaspoon	4	0	15
sun-dried tomatoes in oil, drained, 2 tablespoons	3	1	29
tomato paste, 2 tablespoons	6	1	27
vegetable broth, Pacific Organic, 1 cup	3	0	15

Ingredient and Quantity	Carbs*	Protein*	Calories*
Condiments			
wine, white, dry (used for cooking) (2 ounces or 4 tablespoons, ¼ cup)	2	0	48
Dairy and Cheese			
cottage cheese, ¼ cup (large or small curd)	2	6	55
cream cheese, 2 tablespoons	1	2	101
feta cheese, 1 cubic inch	1	2	45
feta cheese, 1 tablespoon	0	1	25
feta cheese, ½ cup, crumbled	3	11	198
heavy cream, 1 tablespoon	0	0	52
heavy cream, 4 tablespoons (¼ cup)	2	1	205
milk, whole, 1 cup	12	8	149
parmesan, shredded, 1 T	0	2	20
pecorino Romano, grated, 2 teaspoons	0	1	20
sour cream, 1 tablespoon	0	0	23
sour cream, ¼ cup	2	1	111
swiss cheese , 1 slice, 1 oz	2	8	106
yogurt, Greek, ½ cup	4	9	150
yogurt, whole milk, plain, ½ cup	6	4	75
Fruit			
apple, ¼ large	8	0	29
avocado, 1 average	17	4	322
avocado, ¼	4	1	80
blueberries, raw, ¼ cup	5	0	21
cantaloupe, ⅛ medium	6	1	23
lemon juice, ¼ cup (4 tablespoons)	4	0	13
lime juice, 2 tablespoons	3	0	8
orange, medium	16	1	62
orange, small	11	1	45
raisins, golden, ¼ cup, packed	33	1	125
raisins, seedless, ¼ cup, packed	33	1	123
Legumes (Beans) and Grains			
barley, pearled, ½ cup, uncooked	77	10	352
beans, black, cooked, 1 cup	41	15	227

Ingredient and Quantity	Carbs*	Protein*	Calories*
beans, cannellini, canned, Eden, 1 cup	34	12	200
beans, chickpeas, cooked, 1 cup	45	15	265
beans, lentils, cooked, 1 cup	39	18	226
beans, navy, canned, Eden, 1 cup	40	14	220
beans, pinto, cooked, 1 cup	45	15	245
hummus, 1 tablespoon	2	1	23
peanut butter, 2 tablespoons	7	8	190
peanut butter, or almond butter, no sugar added, 2 tablespoons	6	7	190
Meat and Poultry			
bacon, 2 slices, cooked	0	6	92
beef, ground, 90% lean, cooked, 3 ounces	0	24	196
beef, ground, 95% lean, cooked, 3 ounces	0	25	164
beef, steak, flank, cooked, 3 ounces	0	24	173
beef, top sirloin, trimmed, cooked, 3.5 ounces	0	29	212
canadian bacon, 2 ounces	0	11	70
chicken, breast, cooked, roasted, no skin, 3.5 ounces	0	31	165
chicken, dark meat, no skin, roasted, 3.5 ounces	0	27	205
chicken, ground, cooked, 3 ounces	0	20	161
chicken, mixed meat, cooked, 1 cup (about 5 ounces)	0	41	266
chicken, mixed, cooked, 3.5 oz	0	29	185
chicken, white meat, 1 cup (about 5 ounces)	0	43	231
chicken, white meat, cooked, no skin, 1 ounce	0	9	47
egg, 1 average	0	6	80
pork loin, chop, trimmed, cooked, 3.5 ounces	0	28	207
pork loin, trimmed, roasted, 3.5 ounces	0	28	207
pork, ground, cooked, 3 ounces	0	22	252
turkey, breast meat (no skin), roasted, 3.5 ounces	0	30	135

Ingredient and Quantity	Carbs*	Protein*	Calories*
Meat and Poultry			
turkey, dark meat (no skin), roasted, 3.5 ounces	0	28	180
turkey, ground, cooked, 3 ounces	0	23	174
Nuts and Seeds			
almonds, raw, 1 ounce (23 almonds)	6	6	164
pine nuts, ¼ cup	4	5	227
pumpkin seeds, roasted, ⅛ cup	2	4	85
sesame seeds, 1 tablespoon	2	2	52
walnuts, chopped, ⅛ cup	2	2	96
walnuts, raw, 1 ounce (7 whole nuts)	4	4	183
Oils			
canola oil, 1 tablespoon	0	0	124
extra virgin olive oil, 1 tablespoon	0	0	120
extra virgin olive oil, 1 teaspoon	0	0	40
sesame oil, 1 tablespoon	0	0	120
Seafood			
fish, saltwater (grouper, halibut, sea bass, mahi-mahi, orange roughy, cod), average for cooked is 3.5 ounces	0	23	112
halibut, cooked, 4 ounces	0	30	158
salmon, cooked, average of types, 3.5 ounces	0	24	186
shrimp, cooked, 3.5 ounces	0	23	119
tuna, albacore, canned, 2.5 ounce	0	16	120
Vegetables			
artichoke hearts, canned, 2 pieces	7	1	30
asparagus, 4 ounces, 8 to 10 small spears (pen-size)	4	2	22
bell pepper, green, 1 medium	6	1	24
bell pepper, green, ¼ cup, sliced	1	0	6
bell pepper, red or yellow, 1 medium	7	1	37
bell pepper, red or yellow, ¼ cup, sliced	1	0	6
broccoli, 1 cup, raw (3.2 ounces)	6	3	31
cabbage, 1 cup, chopped	5	1	21
cabbage, 1 cup, shredded	4	1	17

Ingredient and Quantity	Carbs*	Protein*	Calories*
carrots, 1 cup, sliced or chopped (2 medium)	12	1	50
carrots, 1 medium	6	0	25
cauliflower, 1 cup, chopped	5	2	27
cauliflower, ½ half of a medium head	15	6	71
celery, 1 cup, chopped	3	1	14
celery, 1 stalk, medium (8")	1	0	6
corn, 1 medium ear, raw	17	3	77
corn, raw, 1 cup	29	5	132
cucumber, peeled, chopped, 1 cup (about 1 small)	3	1	16
cucumber, peeled, medium	4	1	24
cucumber, unpeeled, ½ cup	1.9	0	8
eggplant, 1 cup, cubed	5	1	20
eggplant, 1 ¼ pound	27	5	110
garlic, 1 clove	1	0	4
garlic, 3 cloves	3	1	13
ginger root, 1 tablespoon	1	0	5
green beans, 1 cup, raw	7	2	31
kale, raw, 1 cup, chopped	7	2	34
mushroom, portobello, grilled, 1 cup	5	4	35
mushroom, portobello, raw, 1 cup diced	3	2	19
mushroom, portobello, raw, 100 grams	4	2	22
mushrooms, 100 grams, edible portion	3	3	22
mushrooms, raw, 1 cup, pieces	2	2	15
mushrooms, whole, 4 ounces	4	4	25
onion, 1 cup, chopped	16	2	67
onion, 1 large, 5.3 ounces	15	1	63
onion, 1 medium (2.5-inch in diameter)	11	1	46
onion, 1 small	7	1	28
onion, green, 1 medium	1	0	5
peas, English, ½ cup	11	4	62
peas, green, frozen, ½ cup, cooked	11	4	62
peas, sugar snap (10 pods)	3	1	14
peas, sugar snap, 1 cup, chopped	7	3	41

Ingredient and Quantity	Carbs*	Protein*	Calories*
Vegetables			
romaine, 1 cup, shredded	2	1	8
shallots, chopped, 1 tablespoon	2	0	7
squash, spaghetti, 1 cup	10	1	42
squash, summer, all varieties, 1 cup	4	1	18
summer squash: yellow and zucchini, 1 small (about 1 cup)	4	1	19
sweet potato, baked, small (2.1 ounces)	12	1	54
sweet potatoes, raw, 1 medium (5") —or 1 cup, cubed	26	2	112
tomato, 1 cup, chopped	7	2	32
tomato, 1 medium	5	1	22
tomato, ¼-inch slice	1	0	4

*Note that the numbers in this table are rounded up or down for ease of calculation. (So if the number was 0.5 or higher, we rounded up; if the number was 0.4 or lower, we rounded down.)

Source: USDA Nutritional Database (USDA Food Search for Windows) and CalorieKing (www.calorieking.com).

Appendix C

Wellness 100 Shopping List

Cut out this page, and photocopy it to use as your weekly shopping list and to help you make the best choices at the supermarket. Simply highlight the things that you need, then check them off at the store. You can also download it at http://wellness100.us.

Produce: Buy seasonal, local, and organic as much as possible		feta cheese	
		string cheese	
2 or 3 varieties of salad greens to use in a salad a day		cream cheese (regular, not low-fat)	
		heavy cream (small container)	
celery, carrots, onions, garlic (used in many recipes)		sour cream (small container)	
		whole milk or Greek yogurt	
tomatoes and a variety of fresh vegetables to include in salads as well as to roast, grill, steam, or sauté		**Grains, bread, and beans**	
		100% whole wheat bread	
sweet potato instead of a white potato		whole wheat pita	
parsley and/or cilantro and other fresh herbs as desired		Ezekiel bread	
		corn tortillas (occasionally)	
seasonal fruit		thin sandwich rounds	
avocado		dried or canned beans	
apples and pears (which keep well and have good fiber)		quinoa	
		brown rice	
oranges		**Other**	
lemons and limes		frozen peas	
occasionally: melons, bananas, pineapple (fruit with a high glycemic index)		frozen berries for smoothies, if desired	
Lean meats and seafood: 4 to 6 ounces per portion (buy extra and cook for easy additions to breakfast and lunch)		extra virgin olive oil	
		red-wine vinegar, white-wine vinegar, other flavored vinegars as desired	
steaks or roasts: flank, sirloin, chuck shoulder roast, etc.		pickles and olives	
pork loin chops		canned tuna	
ground beef, 95% lean		no-sugar-added peanut butter	
ground pork, 90% lean (to add to lean, ground turkey breast)		almonds, walnuts, pecans, and other nuts	
		spices as needed	
ground turkey breast		kosher salt	
boneless chicken breasts			
chicken, whole or pieces			
halibut, cod, salmon (wild caught), snapper, mahi mahi, flounder, amber jack, and shrimp are all good choices.			
Eggs, cheese, and dairy			
fresh eggs			
shredded parmesan			

Bibliography

Aberle J, Flitsch J, Beck NA, et al. Genetic variation may influence obesity only under conditions of diet: analysis of three candidate genes. *Molecular Genetics and Metabolism.* November 2008;95(3):188-191.

Abete Itziar PD, Martinez de Morentin B, Martinez JA. Effects of two energy-restricted diets differing in the carbohydrate/protein ratio on weight loss and oxidative changes of obese men. *International Journal of Food Sciences and Nutrition.* January 2009;60(S3):1-13.

Abou-Donia MB, El-Masry EM, Abdel-Rahman AA, McLendon RE, Schiffman SS. Splenda alters gut microflora and increases intestinal p-glycoprotein and cytochrome p-450 in male rats. *Journal of Toxicology and Environmental Health, Part A.* 2008;71:14151429.

Ahima RS. Body fat, leptin, and hypothalamic amenorrhea. *The New England Journal of Medicine.* 2004;351(10):959-962. http://libproxy.ngcsu.edu:2048/login?url=htttp://proquest.umi.com/pqdweb/?did =688524981&sid=5&Fmt=4&clientld=30327&RQT=309&VName=PQD. Accessed March 28, 2010. PQID:6885424981.

Ahmed T, Das SK, Golden JK, et al. Calorie restriction enhances T-cell mediated immune response in adult overweight men and women [abstract]. *The Journals of Gerontology: Series A: Biological sciences and medical sciences.* 2009;64A(11):1107. http://proquest.umi.com/pqdweb?did=1893371991&sid=2&Fmt=2&clie ntld=30327&RQT=309&VName=PQD. Accessed November 8, 2009. PQID:1893371991.

Ahuja KD, Ball MJ. Effects of daily ingestion of chilli on serum lipoprotein oxidation in adult men and women. *British Journal of Nutrition.* 2006;96(2):239-242.

Alaejos MS, Gonzalez V, Afonso AM. Exposure to heterocyclic aromatic amines from the consumption of cooked red meat and its effect on human cancer risk: a review. *Food Additives and Contaminants.* January 2008;25(1):2-24.

Alexandrou E, Herzberg GR, White MD. High-level medium-chain triglyceride feeding and energy expenditure in normal-weight women. *Canadian Journal of Physiology and Pharmacology.* May 2007;85(5):507-513.

Alves JG, Gale CR, Mutrie N, Correia JB, Batty GD. A 6-month exercise intervention among inactive and overweight favela-residing women in Brazil: the Caranguejo exercise trial. *American Journal of Public Health.* January 2009;99(1):76-80. http://libproxy.ngcsu.edu:2048/login?url=http://proquest.umi.com/ pqdweb/?did=1613678991&sid=-1&Fmt=3&clientld=30327&RQT=309&VName=PQD. Accessed March 28, 2010. PQID:1613678991.

Antioxidants; gamma-irradiation reduces antioxidant activity of black pepper. Medical Letter on the CDC & FDA. May 24, 2006:13. http://proquest.umi.com/pqdweb?did=1047457351&Fmt=3&clientld=30327&RQT=3 09&VName=PQD. Accessed November 1, 2009. PQID:1047457351.

Arefhosseini SR, Edwards CA, Malkova D, Higgins S. Effect of advice to increase carbohydrate and reduce fat intake on dietary profile and plasma lipid concentrations in healthy postmenopausal women. *Annals of Nutrition & Metabolism.* 2009;54(2):138-144.

Badman MK, Kennedy AR, Adams AC, Pissios P, Maratos-Flier E. A very low carbohydrate ketogenic diet improves glucose tolerance in ob/ob mice independently of weight loss. *American Journal of Physiology: Endocrinology and metabolism.* November 2009;297(5):e1197.

Barnes L, Romine S. How to keep fruits and veggies fresh. Sparkpeople.com. http://www.sparkpeople.com/ resource/articles_print.asp?i... Accessed October 23, 2011.

Barzilai N, Bartke A. Biological approaches to mechanistically understand the healthy life span extension achieved by calorie restriction and modulation of hormones.*The Journals of Gerontology: Series A: Biological sciences and medical sciences.* February 2009;64A(2):187-192.

Bederman IR, Foy S, Chandramouli V, Alexander JC, Previs SF. Triglyceride synthesis in epididymal adipose tissue. American Society for Biochemistry and Molecular Biology, Inc. 2008. http://ezproxy.pcom.edu:2613/ content/284/10/6101.full. Accessed February 27, 2011.

Bello NT, Guarda AS, Terrillion CE, et al. Repeated binge access to a palatable food alters feeding behavior, hormone profile, and hindbrain c-Fos responses to a test meal in adult male rats [abstract]. *American Journal of Physiology: Regulatory, integrative and comparative physiology.* September 2009;297(3):R622. http://proquest.umi.com/pqdweb?did=1847234681&Fmt=2&clientld=30327&RQT=309&VName=PQD. Accessed November 8, 2009. PQID:1847234681.

Benefits of exercise more than just weight loss. *US Federal News Service, Including US State News.* 2009. http://libproxy.ngcsu.edu:2048/login?url=http://proquest.umi.com/pqdweb/?did=1812185581&sid=-1&Fmt= 3&clientld=30327&RQT=309&VName=PQD. Accessed March 28, 2010. PQID:1812185581.

Bergamini E, Cavallini G, Donati A, Parentini I, Gori Z. The pharmacological intensification of the antiaging effects of calorie restriction (cr) by a physiologic approach. *The Gerontologist.* 2004;44(1):16-17. http://proquest.umi.com/pqdweb?did=918044381&Fmt=3&clientld=30327&RQT=309&VName=PQD.   Accessed November 8, 2009. PQID:918044381.

Berglund ED, Lee-Young RS, Lustig DG, et al. Hepatic energy state is regulated by glucagon receptor signaling in mice. *Journal of Clinical Investigation.* 2009;119(8):2412-2422.

Bergouignan A, Momken I, Schoeller DA, Simon C, Blanc S. Metabolic fate of saturated and monounsaturated dietary fats: the Mediterranean diet revisited from epidemiological evidence to cellular mechanisms. *Progress in Lipid Research.* 2009;48:128-147.

Bhutani S, Varady KA. Nibbling versus feasting: which meal pattern is better for heart disease prevention? *Nutrition Reviews.* 67(10):591-598.

Biolo G, Ciocchi B, Stulle M, et al. Calorie restriction accelerates the catabolism of lean body mass during 2 wk of bed rest [abstract]. *American Journal of Clinical Nutrition.* 2007;86(2):366. http://proquest.umi.com/pqdweb?did=1319841471&Fmt=2&clientld=30327&RQT=309&VName=PQD. Accessed November 8, 2009. PQID: 1319841471.

Blackstone R. Where's the organic beef? How beef gets to your plate. *Alive.* http://www.alive.com/food.

Blending the benefits of flavor and health through herbs and spices. *Nutrition Health Review.* 2008;99:3.

Bliss N. *Real Food All Year: Eating Seasonal Whole Foods for Optimal Health and All-day Energy* [excerpt published by the *California Journal of Oriental Medicine,* ahead of print 2011].

Bocarsly ME, Powell ES, Avena NM, Hoebel BG. High-fructose corn syrup causes characteristics of obesity in rats: increased body weight, body fat and triglyceride levels. *Pharmacology, Biochemistry and Behavior.* 2010;97:101-106.

Bonkowski MS, Rocha JS, Masternak MM, Al Regaiey KA, Bartke A. Targeted disruption of growth hormone receptor interferes with the beneficial actions of calorie restriction [abstract]. *Proceedings of the National Academy of Sciences of the United States of America.* 2006;104(20):7901. http://proquest.umi.com/pqdweb?did=1149836191&Fmt=2&clientld=30327&RQT=309&VName=PQD. Accessed November 8, 2009. PQID:1149836191.

Bouillon R, Norman AW, Lips P, et al. Vitamin D deficiency. *The New England Journal of Medicine.* 2007;357(19):1980. http://libproxy.ngcsu.edu:2048/login?url=http://proquest.umi/com/pqdweb/?dd=1379484881&sid=1Fmt=3&clientld=30327&RQT=309&VName=PQD. Accessed March 14, 2010. PQID:1379484881.

Brader L, Holm L, Mortensen L, et al. Acute effects of casein on postprandial lipemia and incretin responses in type 2 diabetic subjects. *Nutrition, Metabolism & Cardiovascular Diseases.* 2010;20:101-109.

Brugts MP, van Duijn CM, Hofland L J, Witteman JC, Lamberts SWJ, Janssen JA. IGF-I bioactivity in an elderly population. *Diabetes.* 2010;59(2):505-508.

Campbell T Collin, Campbell Thomas M II. *The China Study.* First paperback edition. Dallas, TX: BenBella Books, Inc; 2006.

Can cinnamon combat cholesterol? *Tufts University Health & Nutrition Letter.* 2005;22:11.

Cao Y, Mauger DT, Pelkman CL, et al. Effects of moderate (MF) versus lower fat (LF) diets on lipids and lipoproteins: a meta-analysis of clinical trials in subjects with and without diabetes. *Journal of Clinical Lipidology.* 2009;3:19-32.

Carbohydrate. http://en.wikipedia.org/wiki/Carbohydrate. Accessed March 3, 2011.

Carbohydrates in Wine. http://www.weightlossforall.com/carbohydrates-wine.htm. Accessed September 23, 2009.

Carbs in Wine. http://carb-counter.org/beverages/search/Wine/1400. Accessed September 23, 2009.

Carbs in Wine. http://www.lovetoknow.com/wiki/Carbs_in_Wine. Accessed September 23, 2009.

Carry on, carnitine [abstract}? *University of California, Berkeley, Wellness Letter.* 2009;26(2):2. http://proquest.umi.com/pqdweb?did=1899909571&Fmt=2&clientld=30327&RQT=309&VName=PQD. Accessed November 1, 2009. PQID:1899909571.

Carter CS, Leeuwenburgh C, Daniels M, Foster TC. Influence of calorie restriction on measures of age-related cognitive decline: role of increased physical activity. *The Journals of Gerontology: Series A: Biological sciences and medical sciences.* 2009;64A(8):850-859. http://proquest.umi.com/pqdweb?did=1817036971&Fmt=4&clientld=30327&RQT=309&VName=PQD. Accessed November 8, 2009. PQID:1817036971.

Case Western Reserve University (2011, January 3). Call for truth in trans fats labeling by US FDA: study shows how deceptive food labels lead to increased risk of deadly diseases. *ScienceDaily.* http://www.sciencedaily.com/releases/2011/01/110103110325.htm. Accessed October 23, 2011.

Cheng S, Massaro JM, Fox CS, et al. Adiposity, cardiometabolic risk, and vitamin D status: the Framingham heart study. *Diabetes.* 2010;59(1):242-248. http://libproxy.ngcsu.edu:2048/login?url=http://proquest.umi.com/pqdweb/?did=1958256541&fmt=3&clientld=30327&RQT=309&VName=PQD. Accessed March 14, 2010. PQID:1958256541.

Cheverud JM, Lawson HA, Fawcett GL, et al. Diet-dependent genetic and genomic imprinting effects on obesity in mice. *Obesity Journal.* 2011;19(1):160-170.

Chlebowski RT, Johnson KC, Kooperberg C, et al. Calcium plus vitamin D supplementation and the risk of breast cancer. *Journal of the National Cancer Institute.* 2007;100:1581-1591.

Choi J-S, Choi Y-J, Li J, et al. Dietary flavanoids differentially reduce oxidized LDL-induced apoptosis in human endothelial cells: role of MAPK- and JAK/STAT- signaling. *The Journal of Nutrition.* 2008;138(6):983-990.

Chomentowski P, Dube JJ, Amati F, et al. Moderate exercise attenuates the loss of skeletal muscle mass that occurs with intentional caloric restriction-induced weight loss in older, overweight to obese adults [abstract]. *The Journal of Gerontology: Series A: Biological sciences and medical sciences.* 2009;64A(5):575-581.

Chronic pain; Mayo Clinic study suggests those who have chronic pain may need to assess vitamin D status. *Women's Health Weekly.* 2009;April:92. http://libproxy.ngcsu.edu:2048/login?url=http://proquest.umi.com/pqdweb/?did=1670864681&sid=6&Fmt=3&clientId=30327&RQT=309&VName=PQD. Accessed March 14, 2010. PQID:1670864681.

Claessens M, Calame W, Siemensma AD, van Baak MA, Saris WHM. The effect of different protein hydrolysate/carbohydrate mixtures on postprandial glucagon and insulin responses in healthy subjects. *European Journal of Clinical Nutrition.* 2009;63:48-56.

Claessens M, van Baak MA, Monsheimer S, Saris WHM. The effect of a low-fat, high-protein or high-carbohydrate ad libitum diet on weight loss maintenance and metabolic risk factors. *International Journal of Obesity.* 2009;33:296-304.

Clifton PM, Bastiaans K, Keogh JB. High protein diets decrease total and abdominal fat and improve CVD risk profile in overweight and obese men and women with elevated triacylglycerol. *Nutrition, Metabolism & Cardiovascular Diseases.* 2009;19:548-554.

Cloud J. Eating better than organic. *Time.* http://www.time.com/time/printout/0,8816,1595245,00.html. Accessed October 8, 2011.

Contois JH, McConnell JP, Sethi AA, et al. Apolipoprotein B and cardiovascular disease risk: position statement from the AACC Lipoproteins and Vascular Diseases Division Working Group on Best Practices. *Clinical Chemistry.* 2009;55(3):407-419.

Crinnion WJ. Organic foods contain higher levels of certain nutrients, lower levels of pesticides, and may provide health benefits for the consumer. *Alternative Medicine Review.* 15(1):4-12.

Cromwell WC, Otvos JD. Heterogeneity of low-density lipoprotein particle number in patients with type 2 diabetes mellitus and low-density lipoprotein cholesterol <100 mg/dl. *The American Journal of Cardiology.* December 2006;98(12):1599-1602.

Cromwell WC, Otvos JD, Keyes MJ, et al. LDL particle number and risk of future cardiovascular disease in the Framingham Offspring Study—implications for LDL management. *Journal of Clinical Lipidology.* 2007;1:583-592.

Cronin S. The dual vitamin D pathways: considerations for adequate supplementation. *Nephrology Nursing Journal.* 2010;37(1):19-29. http://libproxy.ngcsu.edu:2048/login?url=http://proquest.umi.com/pqdweb/?did=1971341601&sid=-1&fmt=3&clientId=30327&RQT=309&VName=PQD. Accessed March 14, 2010. PQID: 1971341601.

Crowe TC. Safety of low-carbohydrate diets. *Obesity Reviews.* 2005; 6:235-245.

Cuervo AM. Calorie restriction and aging: the ultimate "cleansing diet." *The Journals of Gerontology: Series A: Biological sciences and medical sciences.* Washington. 2008;63A(6):547-549. http://proquest.umi.co/pqdweb?did=1532864821&Fmt=4&clientId=30327&RQT=309&VName=PQD. Accessed November 8, 2009. PQID: 1532864821.

Culling KS, Neil HAW, Gilbert M, Frayn KN. Effects of short-term low- and high-carbohydrate diets on postprandial metabolism in non-diabetic and diabetic subjects. *Nutrition, Metabolism & Cardiovascular Diseases.* 2009;19:345-351.

Dahlman I, Arner P. Obesity and polymorphisms in genes regulating human adipose tissue. *International Journal of Obesity.* 2007;31:1629-1641.

Dangour AD, Lock K, Hayter A, Aikenhead A, Allen E, Uauy R. Nutrition-related health effects of organic foods: a systematic review. *American Journal of Clinical Nutrition.* 2010;92:203-210.

Danik Suk J, Rifai N, Buring JE, Ridker PM. Lipoprotein(a), measured with an assay independent of apolipoprotein(a) isoform size, and risk of future cardiovascular events among initially healthy women. *Journal of the American Medical Association.* 2006;296(11):1363-1370.

Darwish DS, Wang D, Konat GW, Schreurs BG. Dietary cholesterol impairs memory and memory increases brain cholesterol and sulfatide levels. *Behavioral Neuroscience.* 2010;124(1):115-123.

Dauncey G. Ten reasons why organic food is better. *Common Ground Magazine.* August 2002.

de Jonge L, DeLany JP, Nguyen T, et al. Validation study of energy expenditure and intake during calorie restriction using doubly labeled water and changes in body composition1,2,3 [abstract]. *American Journal of Clinical Nutrition.* 2007;85(1):73. http://proquest.umi.com/pqdweb?did=1200963171&Fmt=2&clientId=30 327&RQT=309&VName=PQD. Accessed November 8, 2009. PQID:1200963171.

Delbridge EA, Prendergast LA, Pritchard JE, Proietto J. One-year weight maintenance after significant weight loss in healthy overweight and obese subjects: does diet composition matter? [abstract]. *American Journal of Clinical Nutrition.* 2009;90(5):1203. http://proquest.umi.com/pqdweb?did=1888973801&Fmt=2&clientId= 30327&RQT=309&VName=PQD. Accessed November 1, 2009. PQID:1888973801.

Demol S, Yackobovitch-Gavan M, Shalitin S, et al. Low-carbohydrate (low & high-fat) versus high-carbohydrate low-fat diets in the treatment of obesity in adolescents. *Acta Paediatrica.* 2009; 98:346-351.

De Natale C, Annuzzi G, Bozzetto L, et al. Effects of a plant-based high-carbohydrate/high-fiber diet versus high-monounsaturated fat/low-carbohydrate diet on postprandial lipids in type 2 diabetic patients. *Diabetes Care.* 2009;32(12):2168-2173.

Dolan LC, Potter SM, Burdock, GA. Evidence-based review on the effect of normal dietary consumption of fructose on development of hyperlipidemia and obesity in healthy, normal weight individuals. *Critical Reviews in Food Science and Nutrition.* 2010;50:53-84.

Dolby Toews V. Hot news about cayenne. *Better Nutrition.* 2007;69(12):22.

Doo Y-C, Han S-J, Lee J-H, et al. Associations among oxidized low-density lipoprotein antibody, C-reactive protein, inerleukin-6, and circulating cell adhesion molecules in patients with unstable angina pectoris[abstract]. *The American Journal of Cardiology.* 2004;93(5):554. http://proquest.umi.com/pdqwe b?did=650302951&sid=11&Fmt=2&clientId=30327&RQT=309&VName=PQD. Accessed November 1, 2009. PQID:650302951.

Downey M. Low calorie longevity. *Better Nutrition.* 2002;64:39-44.

Egert S, Somoza V, Kannemberg F, et al. Influence of three rapeseed oil-rich diets, fortified with α-linolenic acid, eicosapentaenoic acid or docosahexaenoic acid on the composition and oxidizability of low-density lipoproteins: results of a controlled study in healthy volunteers. *European Journal of Clinical Nutrition.* 2007;61:314-325.

Ejaz A, Wu D, Kwan P, Meydani M. Curcumin inhibits adipogenesis in 3T3-L1 adipocytes and angiogenesis and obesity in C57/BL mice. *The Journal of Nutrition.* 2009;139(5):919-928.

El-Arab AM Ezz. A diet rich in leafy vegetable fiber improves cholesterol metabolism in high-cholesterol fed rats. *Pakistan Journal of Biological Sciences.* 2009;12(19):1299-1306.

Elhanany A, Lustman A, Abel R, Attal-Singer J, Vinker S. A low carbohydrate Mediterranean diet improves cardiovascular risk factors and diabetes control among overweight patients with type 2 diabetes mellitus: a 1-year prospective randomized interventions study. *Diabetes, Obesity and Metabolism.* 2010;12:204-209.

Emotional Eating: Overcoming and managing the causes of overeating on MedicineNet. MedicineNet.com. http://www.medicinenet.com/emotional_eating/page2.htm. Accessed September 17, 2009.

Erkkila A, de Mello VDF, Riserus U, Laaksonen DE. Dietary fatty acids and cardiovascular disease: an epidemiological approach. *Progress in Lipid Research.* 2008;47(3):172-187. sciencedirect.com. Accessed March 17, 2011.

Evans L. Foods for radiant skin. *Alive.* http://alive.com/lifestyle.

EWG's 2011 Shopper's Guide to Pesticides in Produce. www.ewg.com. http://www.ewg.org/foodnews/ summary/. Accessed February 22, 2012.

Exercise keeps dangerous visceral fat away year after weight loss, finds University of Alabama at Birmingham study. *US Federal News Service, Including US State News.* October 29, 2009. http://libproxy.ngcsu.edu:2048/ login?url=http://proquest.umi.com/pqdweb/?did=1889372881&sid=-1&Fmt=3&clientId=30327&RQT=309&V Name=PQD. Accessed March 28, 2010. PQID:1889372881.

Faulks SC, Tumer N, Else PL, Hulbert AJ. Calorie restriction in mice: effects on body composition, daily activity, metabolic rate, mitochondrial reactive oxygen species production, and membrane fatty acid composition. *The Journals of Gerontology: Series A: Biological sciences and medical sciences.* 2006;61A(8):781-795. http:// proquest.umi.com/pqdweb?did=1122855271&Fmt=4&clientId=30327&RQT=309&VName=PQD.   Accessed November 8, 2009. PQID:1122855271.

Fernstrom JD. The January issue: Aspartame effects on the brain [editorial]. *European Journal of Clinical Nutrition.* 2009;63:698-699.

Fito M, Guxens M, Corella D, et al. Effect of a traditional Mediterranean diet on lipoprotein oxidation [abstract]. *Archives of Internal Medicine.* 2007;167(11):1195. http://proquest.umi.com/ pqdweb?did=1288139591&sid=11&Fmt-2&clientId=30327&RQT=309&VName=PQD. Accessed November 1, 2009. PQID:1288139591.

Fontana L. Excessive adiposity, calorie restriction, and aging [abstract]. *Journal of the American Medical Association.* 2006;295(13):1577-1578. http://proquest.umi.com/pqdweb?did=1017647341&Fmt=2&clientId=3 0327&RQT=309&VName=PQD. Accessed November 8, 2009. PQID:1017647341.

Fontana L, Klein S. Aging, adiposity, and calorie restriction [abstract]. *Jounal of the American Medical Asoociation.* 2007;297(9):986. http://proquest.umi.com/pqdweb?did=1230875861&Fmt=2&clientId=30327 &RQT=309&VName=PQD. Accessed November 8, 2009. PQID:1230875861.

Fontana L, Villareal DT, Weiss EP, et al. Calorie restriction or exercise: effects on coronary heart disease risk factors. A randomized, controlled trial [abstract]. *American Journal of Physiology: Endocrinology and metabolism.* 2007;293(1):E197. http://proquest.umi.com/pqdweb?did=1302065041&Fmt=2&clientId=30327 &RQT=309&VName=PQD. Accessed November 8, 2009. PQID:1302065041.

Foster GD, Wyatt HR, Hill JO, et al. Weight and metabolic outcomes after 2 years on a low-carbohydrate versus low-fat diet. *Annals of Internal Medicine.* 2010;153:147-157.

Foster-Powell K, Holt SHA, Brand-Miller JC. International table of glycemic index and glycemic load values: 2002. *American Journal of Clinical Nutrition.* 2002;76:5-56.

Fuhrman B, Rosenblat M, Hayek T, Coleman R, Aviram M. Ginger extract consumption reduces plasma cholesterol, inhibits LDL oxidation and attenuates development of atherosclerosis in atherosclerotic, apolipoprotein e-deficient mice. *The Journal of Nutrition.* 2000;130(5):1124-1130.

Fung TT, van Dam RM, Hankinson SE., et al. Low-carbohydrate diets and all-cause and cause-specific mortality. *Annals of Internal Medicine.* 2010;153:289-298.

Gaffney-Stomberg E, Insogna KL, Rodriguez NR, Kerstetter JE. Increasing dietary protein requirements in elderly people for optimal muscle and bone health. *Journal of the American Geriatrics Society.* 2009;57(6):1073-1079.

Gamma-irradiation reduces antioxidant activity of black pepper. *Medical Letter on the CDC & FDA.* 2006;13.

Garrido-Sanchez L, Garcia-Fuentes E, Rojo-Martinez G, Cardona F, Soriguer F, Tinahones FJ. Inverse relation between levels of anti-oxidized-LDL antibodies and eicosapentaeonic acid (EPA). *British Journal of Nutrition.* 2008;100:585-589.

Giugliano D, Ceriello A, Esposito K. The effects of diet on inflammation. *Journal of the American College of Cardiology.* 2006;48(4):677-685.

Glycemic index and glycemic load for 100+ foods. http://www.health.harvard.edu/newsweek/Glycemic_index_ and_glycemic_load_for_100_foods.htm.

Glycemic Index. BL Publications and NHL Ministries. http://www.blpublications.com/htlml/body_gycemicindex. html. Accessed October 3, 2009.

Gray J, Griffin B. Eggs and dietary cholesterol—dispelling the myth. British Nutrition Foundation *Nutrition Bulletin.* 2009;34:66-70.

Greene CM, Waters D, Clark RM, Contois JH, Fernandez ML. Plasma LDL and HDL characteristics and carotenoid content are positively influenced by egg consumption in an elderly population. *Nutrition & Metabolism.* 2006;3:6.

Grifantini K. Understanding pathways of calorie restriction: a way to prevent cancer? *Journal of the National Cancer Institute News.* 2008;100(9):619-621.

Grun F, Blumberg B. Minireview: the case for obesogens. *Molecular Endocrinology.* 2009;23(8):1127-1134.

Guarente L. Sirtuins as potential targets for metabolic syndrome. *NATURE.* 2006;444:868-874.

Guart A, Bono-Blay F, Borrell A, Lacorte S. Migration of plasticizers phthalates, bisphenol A and alkylphenols from plastic containers and evaluation of risk. *Food Additives and Contaminants.* 2011;28(5):676-685.

Habib P, Scrocco JD, Terek M, Vanek V, Mikolich JR. Effects of bariatric surgery on inflammatory, functional and structural markers of coronary atherosclerosis [abstract]. *The American Journal of Cardiology.* 2009;104(9):1251. http://proquest.umi.com/pqdweb?did=1884962661&Fmt=2&clientId=30327&RQT=309& VName=PQD. Accessed November 1, 2009. PQID:1884962661.

Hagopian K, Harper M-E, Ram JJ, et al. Long-term calorie restriction reduces proton leak and hydrogen peroxide production in liver mitochondria [abstract]. *American Journal of Physiology: Endocrinology and metabolism.* 2005;51(1):E674. http://proquest.umi.com/pqdweb?did=830558601&Fmt=2&clientId=30327& RQT=309&VName=PQD. Accessed November 8, 2009. PQID:830558601.

Harman NL, Leeds AR, Griffin BA. Increased dietary cholesterol does not increase plasma low density lipoprotein when accompanied by an energy-restricted diet and weight loss. *European Journal of Nutrition.* 2008;47:287-293.

Hassanali Z, Ametaj BN, Field CJ, Proctor SD, Vine DF. Dietary supplementation of n-3 PUFA reduces weight gain and improves postprandial lipaemia and the associated inflammatory response in the obese JCR:LA-cp rat. *Diabetes, Obesity and Metabolism.* 2010;12:139-147.

Hatfield H. Emotional eating: feeding your feelings. WebMD.com. http://www.webmd.com/diet/features/ emotional-eating-feeding-your-feelings. Accessed September 17, 2009.

Heber D. Phytochemicals beyond antioxidation [expanded abstract]. *The Journal of Nutrition.* 2004;134(11):3175S-3176S.

Height and Weight Charts. http://www.healthchecksystems.com/heightweightchart.html. Accessed September 23, 2009.

Heilbronn LK, de Jonge L, Frisard MI, et al. Effect of 6-month calorie restriction on biomarkers of longevity, metabolic adaptation, and oxidative stress in overweight individuals: a randomized controlled trial [abstract]. *Journal of the American Medical Association.* 2006;295(13):1539-1548. http://proquest.umi.com/pqdweb?did=1017647241&Fmt=2&clientId=30327&RQT=309&VName=PQD. Accessed November 8, 2009. PQID:1017647241.

Hernandez T, Sutherland JP, Wolfe P, et al. Lack of suppression of circulating free fatty acids and hypercholesterolemia during weight loss on a high-fat, low-carbohydrate diet. *American Journal of Clinical Nutrition.* 2010;91:578-585.

Hession M, Rolland C, Kulkarni U, Wise A, Broom J. Systematic review of randomized controlled trials of low-carbohydrate vs. low-fat/low-calorie diets in the management of obesity and its comorbidities. *Obesity Reviews.* 2008;10:36-50.

Higashi Y, Sukhanov S, Parthasarathy S, Delafontaine P. The ubiquitin ligase Nedd4 mediates oxidized low-density lipoprotein-induced downregulation of insulin-like growth factor-1 receptor [abstract]. *American Journal of Physiology: Heart and circulatory physiology.* 2008;295(4):H1684. http://proquest.umi.com/pqdweb?did=1572471361&sid=10&Fmt=2&clientId=30327&RQT=309&VName=PQD. Accessed November 8, 2009. PQID:1572471361.

Hintzpeter B, Mensink GBM, Thierfelder W, Muller MJ, Scheidt-Nave C. Vitamin D status and health correlates among German adults. *European Journal of Clinical Nutrition.* 2008;62:1079-1089.

Hlebowicz J, Hlebowicz A, Lindstedt S, et al. Effects of 1 and 3 g cinnamon on gastric emptying, satiety, and postprandial blood glucose, insulin, glucose-dependent insulinotropic polypeptide, glucagon-like peptide 1, and ghrelin concentrations in healthy subjects [abstract]. *American Journal of Clinical Nutrition.* 2009;89(3):815. http://proquest.umi.com/pqdweb?did=1651765231&Fmt=2&clientId=30327&RQT=309&VName=PQD. Accessed November 1, 2009. PQID: 1651765231.

Hodgson JM, Lee YP, Puddey IB, et al. Effects of increasing dietary protein and fibre intake with lupin on body weight and composition and blood lipids in overweight men and women. *International Journal of Obesity.* 2010;341086-1094.

Holick MF. Vitamin D: importance in the prevention of cancers, type 1 diabetes, heart disease, and osteoporosis [abstract]. *The American Journal of Clinical Nutrition.* 2004;70(3):362. http://libproxy.ngcsu.edu:2048/login?url=http://proquest.umi.com/pqdweb/?did=679592211&sid=1&Fmt=2&clientId=30327&RQT=309&VName=PQD. Accessed March 14, 2010. PQID:679592211.

Holick MF. Vitamin D deficiency medical progress. *The New England Journal of Medicine.* 2007;357(3)266. http://libproxy.ngcsu.edu:2048/login?url=http://proquest.umi.com/pqdweb/?did=1307022581&sid=1&Fmt=4&clientId=30327&RQT=309&VName=PQD. Accessed March 14, 2010. PQID:1307022581.

Holven KB, Scholz H, Halvorsen B, Aukrust P, Ose L, Nenseter MS. Hyperhomocysteinemic subjects have enhanced expression of lectin-like oxidized LDL receptor-1 in mononuclear cells. *The Journal of Nutrition.* 2003;133(11):3588-3591.

Houston MC, Fazio S, Chilton FH, et al. Nonpharmacologic treatment of dyslipidemia. *Progress in Cardiovascular Diseases.* 2009;52:61-94.

Hu FB, Stampfer MJ, Manson JE, et al. Dietary saturated fats and their food sources in relation to the risk of coronary heart disease in women. *American Journal of Clinical Nutrition.* 1999;70:1001-1008. http://www.ajcn.org at Philadelphia College of Osteopathic Medicine. Accessed March 17, 2011.

Hulley S, Grady D. Postmenopausal hormone treatment. *Journal of the American Medical Association.* 2009; 301(23):2493.

Humphries P, Pretorius E, Naudé H. Direct and indirect cellular effects of aspartame on the brain. *European Journal of Clinical Nutrition.* 2008;62(4):451-462.

Ikeno Y, Hubbard GB, Lee S, et al. Reduced incidence and delayed occurrence of fatal neoplastic diseases in growth hormone receptor/binding protein knockout mice. *The Journals of Gerontology.* 2009;64A:522-529.

Jakobsen MU, Overvad K, Dyerberg J, Schroll M, Heitmann BL. Dietary fat and risk of coronary heart disease: possible effect modification by gender and age. *American Journal of Epidemiology.* 2004;196:141-149.

Jenkins DJA, Chiavaroli L, Wong JMW, et al. Adding monounsaturated fatty acids to a dietary portfolio of cholesterol-lowering foods in hypercholesterolemia. *Canadian Medical Association Journal.* 2010;182(18):1961-1967.

Jennings K-A. 3 health reasons to cook with cast-iron. Food on Shine. shine.yahoo.com. http://shine.yahoo.com/channel/food/3-heath-reasons-to-. Accessed October 8, 2011.

Johnston N, Jernberg T, Lagerqvist B, Siegbahn A, Wallentin L. Improved identification of patients with coronary artery disease by the use of new lipid and lipoprotein biomarkers [abstract]. *The American Journal of Cardiology.* 2006;97(5):640. http://proquest.umi.com/pqdweb?did=1010285141&sid=11&Fmt=2&clientId=30327&RQT=309&VName=PQD. Accessed November 8, 2009. PQID:1010285141.

Kala A, Prakash J. The comparative evaluation of the nutrient composition and sensory attributes of four vegetables cooked by different methods. *International Journal of Food Science and Technology.* 2006;41:163-171.

Kathiresan S, Otvos JD, Sullivan LM, et al. Increased small low-density lipoprotein particle number: a prominent feature of the metabolic syndrome in the Framingham heart study. *Journal of the American Heart Association.* 2006;113:20-29.

Kelbe A. Spices and type 2 diabetes. *Nutrition and Food Science.* 2005;35(2):81-87.

Kim J-Y, Yang Y-H, Kim C-N, et al. Effects of very-low-carbohydrate (horsemeat or beef-based) diets and restricted feeding on weight gain, feed and energy efficiency, as well as serum levels of cholesterol, triacylglycerol, glucose, insulin and ketone bodies in adult rats. *Annals of Nutritional & Metabolism.* 2008;53:260-267.

Kim J-Y, Yang Y-H, Kim C-N, Lee C-E, Kim K-I. Effects of very-low-carbohydrate (horsemeat- or beef-based) diets and restricted feeding on weight gain, feed and energy efficiency, as well as serum levels of cholesterol, triacylglycerol, glucose, insulin and ketone bodies in adult rats [abstract]. *Annals of Nutrition & Metabolism.* 2009;53(3-4):260-267. http://libproxy.northgeorgia.edu/login?url=http://proquest.umi.com/pqdweb/?did=1649813151&sid=9&Fmt=2&clientId=30327&RQT=309&VName=PQD. Accessed October 24, 2010. PQID:1649813151.

Kowalsky GB, Byfield FJ, Levitan I. oxLDL facilitates flow-induced realignment of aortic endothelial cells [abstract]. *American Journal of Physiology.* 2008;295(2):C332. http://proquest.umi.com/pqdweb?did=1530331611&sid=11&Fmt=2&clientId=30327&RQT=309&VName=PQD. Accessed November 1, 2009. PQID:1530331611.

Kummerow FA. The negative effects of hydrogenated trans fats and what to do about them. *Atherosclerosis.* 2009;205(2):458-465.

Lapointe A, Goulet J, Couillard C, Lamarche B, Lemiuex S. A nutritional intervention promoting the Mediterranean food pattern is associated with a decrease in circulating oxidized LDL particles in healthy women from the Quebec City metropolitan area. *The Journal of Nutrition.* 2005;135(3):410-415.

Larson-Meyer DE, Heilbronn LK, Redman LM, et al. Effect of calorie restriction with or without exercise on insulin sensitivity, β-cell function, fat cell size, and ectopic lipid in overweight subjects. *Diabetes Care.* 2006;29(6):1337-1344.

Lau BHS. Suppression of LDL oxidation by garlic compounds is a possible mechanism of cardiovascular health benefit. *The Journal of Nutrition.* 2006;136(3S):765S-768S.

LaValle James B, Yale Stacy Lundin. *Cracking the metabolic code: 9 keys to optimal health.* Laguna Beach, CA: Basic Health Publications, Inc; 2004.

Leavitt SB. Vitamin D for chronic pain. *Practical Pain Management.* July/August 2008:24-42.

Lee A, Griffin B. Dietary cholesterol, eggs, and coronary heart disease risk in perspective. British Nutrition Foundation *Nutrition Bulletin.* 2006;31:21-27.

Lee TYA, Li Z, Zerlin A, Heber D. Effects of dihydrocapsiate on adaptive and diet-induced thermogenesis with a high protein very low calorie diet: a randomized control trial. *Nutrition & Metabolism.* 2010;7:78.

Leventis P, Patel S. Clinical aspects of vitamin D in the management of rheumatoid arthritis. *Rheumatology.* 2008;47:1617-1621.

Lin C-TJ, Yen ST. Knowledge of dietary fats among US consumers. *Journal of the American Dietetic Association.* 2010;110(4):613-618.

Lopez-Lluch G, Hunt N, Jones B, et al. Calorie restriction induces mitochondrial biogenesis and bioenergetic efficiency [abstract]. *Proceedings of the National Academy of Sciences of the United States of America.* Washington. 2006;103(6):1768. http://proquest.umi.com/pqdweb?did=994163001&Fmt=2&clientId=30327&RQT=309&VName=PQD. Accessed November 8, 2009. PQID:994163001.

Lopez-Miranda J, Badimon L, Bonanome A, et al. Monounsaturated fat and cardiovascular risk. *Nutrition Reviews.* 2006;64(10):S2-S12.

Lopez-Oliva E, Nus M, Agis-Torres A, et al. Growth hormone improves lipoprotein concentration and arylesterase activity in mice with an atherogenic lipid profile induced by lactalbumin. *British Journal of Nutrition.* 2009;101:510-518.

Lowcarbezine! What are good carbs? http://www.lowcarbohydrate.net/httblog/archives/000148.html. Accessed October 3, 2009.

Lunn J. Monounsaturates in the diet. *Nutrition Bulletin.* 2007;32:378-391.

Lunn J, Theobald HE. The health effects of dietary unsaturated fatty acids. *Nutrition Bulletin.* 2006;31:178-224.

Magkos F, Arvaniti F, Zampelas A. Organic food: buying more safety or just peace of mind? A critical review of the literature. *Critical Reviews in Food Science and Nutrition.* 2006;46:23-56.

Magnuson BA, Burdock GA, Doull J, et al. Aspartame: a safety evaluation based on current use levels, regulations, and toxicological and epidemiological studies. *Critical Reviews in Toxicology.* 2007;37:629-727.

Maidment C, Dyson A, Haysom I. A study into the antimicrobial effects of cloves (syzgium aromaticum) and cinnamon (cinnamomum zeylanicum) using disc-diffusion assay. *Nutrition & Food Science.* 2006;36(4):225-230.

Manjunatha H, Srinivasan, K. Protective effect of dietary curcumin and capsaicin on induced oxidation of low-density lipoprotein, iron-induced hepatotoxicity and carrageenan-induced inflammation in experimental rats [abstract]. *The FEBS Journal*. 2006;273(19):4528. http://proquest.umi.com/pqdweb?did=1129683921&sid=11&Fmt=2&clientId=30327&RQT=309&VName=PQD. Accessed November 1, 2009. PQID:1129683921

Mann JI. Diet and risk of coronary heart disease and type 2 diabetes. *The Lancet*. 2002;360:783-789.

Martin CK, Anton SD, York-Crowe E, et al. Empirical evaluation of the ability to learn a calorie counting system and estimate portion size and food intake. *The British Journal of Nutrition*. 2007;98(2):439-444.

Masella R, Vari R, D'Archivio M, et al. Extra virgin olive oil biophenols inhibit cell-mediated oxidation of LDL by increasing the mRNA transcription of glutathione-related enzymes. *The Journal of Nutrition*. 2004;134(4):785-791.

Masternak MM, Panici JA, Bonkowski MS, Hughes LF, Bartke A. Insulin sensitivity as a key mediator of growth hormone actions on longevity. *The Journals of Gerontology Series A: Biological sciences and medical sciences* . 2009;64A:516-521.

Mathur A, Al-Azzawi HH, Lu D, et al. Steatocholecystitis: the influence of obesity and dietary carbohydrates. *Journal of Surgical Research*. 2008;147:290-297.

Mauvoisin D, Mounier C. Hormonal and nutritional regulation of SCD1 gene expression. *Biochimie*. 2011;93:78-86.

Mayo Clinic Staff. Organic foods: are they safer? More nutritious? December 3, 2011. http://www.mayoclinic.com/health/organic-food/NU00255. Accessed October 18, 2011.

McCarter R, Mejia W, Ikeno Y, et al. Plasma glucose and the action of calorie restriction on aging. *The Journals of Gerontology: Series A: Biological sciences and medical sciences*. 2007;62A(10):1059-1070. http://proquest.umi.com/pqdweb?did=1373549851&Fmt=4&clientId=30327&RQT=309&VName=PQD. Accessed November 8, 2009. PQID:1373549851.

McCurdy CE, Davidson RT, Cartee GD. Calorie restriction increases the ratio of phosphatidylinositol 3-kinase catalytic to regulatory subunits in rat skeletal muscle. *American Journal of Physiology: Endocrinology and metabolism*. 2005;51(5):E996. http://proquest.umi.com/pqdweb?did=832217031&Fmt=2&clientId=30327&RQT=309&VName=PQD. Accessed November 8, 2009. PQID:832217031.

McGill AEJ. The potential effects of demands for natural and safe foods on global food security. *Trends in Food and Science Technology*. 2009;20:402-406.

McKiernan SH, Tuen VC, Baldwin K, et al. Adult-onset calorie restriction delays the accumulation of mitochondrial enzyme abnormalities in aging rat kidney tubular epithelial cells [abstract]. *American Journal of Physiology: Renal Physiology*. 2007;292(6):F1751. http://proquest.umi.com/pqdweb?did=1282599511&Fmt=2&clientId=30327&RQT=309&VName=PDQ. Accessed November 8, 2009. ProQuest document ID:1282599511

McLaughlin T, Carter S, Lamendola C, et al. Clinical efficacy of two hypocaloric diets that vary in overweight patients with type 2 diabetes. *Diabetes Care*. 2007;30(7):1877-1879.

Mignone LI, Giovannucci E, Newcomb PA, et al. Meat consumption, heterocyclic amines, NAT2, and the risk of breast cancer. *Nutrition and Cancer*. 2009;61(1):36-46.

Mofor CT, Medjida NML, Kuate JB, Kana SMM, Zollo PHA. Antioxidant capacity of four mixtures of spices and condiments used in Africa [abstract]. *Journal of Nutrition Education and Behavior.* 2009; 41(4S):S45. http://proquest.umi.com/pqdweb?did=1777671781&Fmt=2clientId=30327&RQT=309&VName=PQD.   Accessed November 1, 2009. PQID:1777671781.

Moon J-Y, Kwon HM, Kwon SW, et al. Lipoprotein(a) and LDL particle size are related to the severity of coronary artery disease. *European Journal of Clinical Nutrition*. 2007;108:282-289.

Moreno JA, Lopez-Miranda J, Perez-Martinez P, et al. A monounsaturated fatty acid-rich diet reduces macrophage uptake of plasma oxidised low-density lipoprotein in healthy young men. *British Journal of Nutrition*. 2008;100:569-575.

Morrison C. Interaction between exercise and leptin in the treatment of obesity. *Diabetes*. 2008;57(3):534-535. http://libproxy.ngcsu.edu:2048/login?url=http://proquest.umi.com/pqdweb/?did=1453078731&sid=-1&Fmt=3&clientId=30327&RQT=309&VName=PQD. Accessed March 28, 2010. PQID:1453078731.

Mozaffarian D, Cao H, King IB, et al. Circulating palmitoleic acid and risk of metabolic abnormalities and new-onset diabetes. *American Journal of Clinical Nutrition*. 2010;92(6):1350-1358.

Muller-Ehmsen J, Braun D, Schneider T, et al. Decreased number of circulating progenitor cells in obesity: beneficial effects of weight reduction. *European Heart Journal*. 2008;29:1560-1568.

Natoli S, Markovic T, Lim D, Noakes M, Kostner K. Unscrambling the research: eggs, serum cholesterol and coronary heart disease. *Nutrition & Dietetics*. 2007;64:105-111.

Nauert R. Reduce emotional eating. *Psych Central News*. http://psychcentral.com/news/2009/08/14/reduce-emtional-eating/7762.html. Accessed September 17, 2009.

Naukkarinen J, Surakka I, Pietilainen KH, et al. Use of genome-wide expression data to mine the "gray zone" of GWA studies leads to novel candidate obesity genes. *Public Library of Science Genetics*. 2010;6(6): 1-9.

Nelson-Dooley C, Kaplan S, Bralley JA. Migraines and mood disorders: nutritional and dietary intervention based on laboratory testing. *Alternative Therapies.* 2009;15(5):56-60.

Nettleton JA, Steffen LM, Loehr LR, Rosamond WD, Folsom AR. Incident heart failure is associated with lower whole-grain intake and greater high-fat dairy and egg intake in the atherosclerosis risk in communities (ARIC) study. *Journal of the American Dietetic Association.* 2008;108:1881-1887.

Neuroactive steroid. Wikipedia.org. http://en.wikipedia.org/w/index.php?title=Neuroactive_steroid&printable =yes. Accessed August 19, 2010.

Nicklas BJ, Wan X, You T, et al. Effect of exercise on abdominal fat loss during calorie restriction in overweight and obese postmenopausal women: a randomized, controlled trial [abstract]. *American Journal of Clinical Nutrition.* 2009;89(4):1043. http://proquest.umi.com/pqdweb?did=1666109751&Fmt=2&clientId=30327&R QT=309&VName=PQD. Accessed November 8, 2009. PQID:1666109751.

Ninfali P, Mea Gloria, GS, Rocchi M, Macchiocca M. Antioxidant capacity of vegetables, spices and dressings relevant to nutrition. *British Journal of Nutrition.* 2005;93:257-266.

Njike V, Faridi Z, Dutta S, Gonzalez-Simon A, Katz DL. Daily egg consumption in hyperlipidemic adults—effects on endothelial function and cardiovascular risk. *Nutrition Journal.* 2010;9:28.

Noakes M, Foster PR, Keogh JB, James AP, Mamo JC, Clifton PM. Comparison of isocaloric very low carbohydrate/high saturated fat and high carbohydrate/low saturated fat diets on body composition and cardiovascular risk. *Nutrition and Metabolism.* 2006;3:7.

Nonstick cookware emits toxic chemicals. *New Vegetarian & Natural Health.* Summer 2001/2002:12.

Oliver MF. It is more important to increase the intake of unsaturated fats than to decrease the intake of saturated fats: evidence from clinical trials relating to ischemic heart disease. *American Journal of Clinical Nutrition.* 1997;66(suppl):980S-986S.

Omura Y, Lee AY, Beckman SL, et al. 177 cardiovascular risk factors, classified in 10 categories, to be considered in the prevention of cardiovascular diseases: an update of the original 1982 article containing 96 risk factors. *Acupuncture & Electro-Therapeutics Research.* 1996;21(1):21-76.

Ortolani C, Pastorello EA. Food allergies and food intolerances. *Best Practice & Research Clinical Gastroenterology.* 2006;20(3):467-483.

Owen OE, Kavle E, Owen RS, Polansky M, Caprio S, Mozzoli MA, et al. A reappraisal of caloric requirements in healthy women. *The American Journal of Clinical Nutrition.* 1986;44:1-19.

Papakonstantinou E, Zampelas A. The effect of dietary protein intake on coronary heart disease risk. British Nutrition Foundation *Nutrition Bulletin.* 2008;333:287-297.

Park S-H, Lee K-S, Park H-Y. Dietary carbohydrate intake is associated with cardiovascular disease risk in Korean: analysis of the third Korea National Health and Nutrition Examination Survey (KNHANES III). *International Journal of Cardiology.* 2010;139(3):234-240.

Park Y, Lim J, Kwon Y, Lee J. Correlation of erythrocyte fatty acid composition and dietary intakes with markers of atherosclerosis in patients with myocardial infarction. *Nutrition Research.* 2009;29(6):391-396.

Peregrin T. Bone up on calorie restriction diet [abstract]. *Journal of the American Dietetic Association.* 2008;108(12):1977. http://proquest.umi.com/pqdweb?did=1613057141&Fmt=2&clientId=30327&RQT=309&V Name=PQD. Accessed November 8, 2009. PQID:1613057241.

Pieke B, von Eckardstein A, Gulbahce E, et al. Treatment of hypertriglyceridemia by two diets rich either in unsaturated fatty acids or in carbohydrates: effects on lipoprotein subclasses, lipolytic enzymes, lipid transfer proteins, insulin and leptin. *International Journal of Obesity.* 2000;24:1286-1296.

Power L. Biotype diets system®:blood types and food allergies. *Journal of Nutritional & Environmental Medicine.* 2007;16(2):125-135.

Puska P. Fat and heart disease: yes we can make a change–the case of North Karelia (Finland). *Annals of Nutritional Metabolism* 2009;54(suppl 1):33-38.

Radhika G, Ganesan A, Sathya RM, Sudha V, Mohan V. Dietary carbohydrates, glycemic load and serum high-density lipoprotein cholesterol concentrations among South Indian adults. *European Journal of Clinical Nutrition.* 2009;63:412-420.

Radulescu A, Gannon MC, Nuttall FQ. The effect on glucagon, glucagon-like peptide-1, total and acyl-ghrelin of dietary fats ingested with and without potato. *Journal of Clinical Endocrinology and Metabolism.* 2010;95:3385-3391.

Raman A, Ramsey JJ, Kemnitz J, et al. Influences of calorie restriction and age on energy expenditure in the rhesus monkey [abstract]. *The American Journal of Physiology: Endocrinology and metabolism.* 2007;292(1):E101. http://proquest.umi.com/pqdweb?did=1191032371&Fmt=2&clientId=30327&RQT=309&V Name=PQD. Accessed November 8, 2009. PQID:1191032371.

Redman LM, Rood J, Anton SD, et al. Calorie restriction and bone health in young, overweight individuals [abstract]. *Archives of Internal Medicine.* 2008;168(17):1859. http://proquest.umi.com/pqdweb?did=15667 01041&Fmt=2&clientId=30327&RQT=309&VName=PQD. Accessed November 8, 2009. PQID:1566701041.

Reed J, Frazão E, Itskowitz R. How expensive are fruits and vegetables anyway? *Amber Waves: The Economics of Food, Farming, Natural Resources, and Rural America.* July 2004. http://www.ers.usda.gov/AmberWaves/september05/findings/FruitVeg.htm. Accessed September 5, 2011.

Roberts R, Bickerton AS., Fielding BA, et al. Reduced oxidation of dietary fat after a short term high-carbohydrate diet. *American Journal of Clinical Nutrition.* 2008;87:824-31.

Rodriguez-Moran M, Guerrero-Romero F, Rascon-Pacheco RA. Dietary factors related to the increase of cardiovascular risk factors in traditional Tepehuanos communities from Mexico. A 10 year follow-up study. *Nutrition, Metabolism and Cardiovascular Diseases.* 2009;19(6):409-416. sciencedirect.com. Accessed February 27, 2011.

Ruxton C. Recommendations for the use of eggs in the diet. *Nursing Standard.* 2010;24(37):47-55.

Saraswat M, Yadagiri RP, Muthenna P, Bhanuprakash RP. Prevention of non-enzymic glycation of proteins by dietary agents: prospects for alleviating diabetic complications [abstract]. *The British Journal of Nutrition.* 2009;101(11):1714. http://proquest.umi.com/pqdweb?did=1801523151&Fmt=2&clientId=30327&RQT=309&VName=PQD. Accessed November 1, 2009. PQID:1801523151.

Schmidt Michael A. *Brain-building nutrition.* 3rd ed. Berkeley, CA: Frog, Ltd; 2007.

Scott E, About.com. Stress and emotional eating: what causes emotional eating? About.com. http://stress.about.com/od/unhealthybehaviors/a/eating.htm. Accessed September 17, 2009.

Scotter MJ, Castle L. Chemical interactions between additives in foodstuffs: a review. *Food Additives and Contaminants.* 2004;21(2):93-124.

Seale P, Lazar MA. Brown fat in humans: turning up the heat on obesity. *Diabetes.* 2009;58(7):1482-1484. http://libproxy.ngcsu.edu:2048/login?url=htpp://proquest.umi.com/pqdweb/?did=1799979711&sid=-1&Fmt=4&clientId=30327&RQT=309&VName=PQD. Accessed March 28, 2010.PQID:1799979711.

Sharman MJ, Gomez AL, Kraemer WJ, et al. Very low-carbohydrate and low-fat diets affect fasting lipids and postprandial lipemia differently in overweight men. *The Journal of Nutrition.* 2004;134(4):880-885.

Sharratt L. Genetically engineered foods. Past, present and future. *Alive.* http://www.alive.com/lifestyle.

Sies H, Stahl W, Sevanian A. Nutritional, dietary, and postprandial oxidative stress. *The Journal of Nutrition.* 2005; 135(5): 969-972.

Sik KW, Sok LY, Hun CS, et al. Berberine improves lipid dysregulation in obesity by controlling central and peripheral AMPK activity. *American Journal of Physiology: Endocrinology and metabolism.* 2009;296(4):E812.

Simeons ATW. *Pounds and Inches.* 1954. http://greenvalleyspa.com/weight-loss-program/information-gallery/pounds-and-inches. Accessed July 6, 2009.

Sinatra S. 10 must-know facts about cholesterol. *Heart, Health & Nutrition.* August 2008:4.

Sinatra S. Let's clear up the cholesterol confusion once and for all. *Heart, Health & Nutrition.* August 2008.

Singletary K. Cinnamon: overview of health benefits [abstract]. *Nutrition Today.* 2008;43(6):263. http://proquest.umi.com/pqd?did=1624485511&Fmt=2&clientId=30327&RQT=309&VName=PQD. Accessed November 1, 2009. PQID:1624485511.

Siri-Tarino PW, Sun Q, Hu FB, Krauss RM. Meta-analysis of prospective cohort studies evaluating the association of saturated fat with cardiovascular disease. *American Journal of Clinical Nutrition.* 2010;91:353-546. http://www.ajcn.org at Philadelphia College of Osteopathic Medicine. Accessed March 17, 2011.

Skeaff MC, Thoma C, Mann J, Chisholm A, Williams S, Richmond K. Isocaloric substitution of plant sterol-enriched fat spread for carbohydrate-rich foods in a low-fat, fibre-rich diet decreases plasma low-density lipoprotein cholesterol and increases high-density lipoprotein concentrations. *Nutrition, Metabolism & Cardiovascular Diseases.* 2005;15:337-344.

Smith SR. A look at the low-carbohydrate diet. *The New England Journal of Medicine.* 2009;361(23):2286.

Soffritti M, Belpoggi F, Tibaldi E, Esposti DD, Lauriola M. Life span exposure to low doses of aspartame beginning during prenatal life increases cancer effects in rats. *Environmental Health Perspectives.* 2007;115(9):1293-1297.

Steinberg D. Statins, the cholesterol controversy, and preventive cardiology [editorial]. *The Lancet.* 2009;374:517-518.

Stocker R, Keaney JF Jr. Role of oxidative modifications in atherosclerosis [abstract]. *Physiological Reviews.* 2004;84(4):1381. http://proquest.umi.com/pqdweb?did=739431281&sid=11&Fmt=2&clientId=30327&RQT=309&VName=PQD. Accessed November 1, 2009. PQID:739431281.

Stoernell CK, Tangney CC, Rockway SW., Short-term changes in lipoprotein subclasses and c-reactive protein levels of hypertriglyceridemic adults on low-carbohydrate and low-fat diets. *Nutrition Research.* 2008;28:443-449.

Stover PJ, Caudill MA. Genetic and epigenetic contributions to human nutrition and health: managing genome-diet interactions. *Journal of the American Dietetic Association.* 2008;108:1480-1487.

Straznicky NE, Lambert EA, Nestel PJ, et al. Sympathetic neural adaptation to hypocaloric diet with or without exercise training in obese metabolic syndrome subjects. *Diabetes.* 2010;59(1):71-80. http://libproxy.ngcsu.

edu:2048/login?url=http://proquest.umi.com/pqdweb/?did=1958256381&sid=-1&Fmt=4&clientId=30327&RQT=309&VName=PQD. Accessed March 28, 2010. PQID:1958256381.

Straznicky NE, Lambert GW, McGrane MT, et al. Weight loss may reverse blunted sympathetic neural responsiveness to glucose ingestion in obese subjects with metabolic syndrome. *Diabetes.* 2009;58(5):1126-1132. http://libproxy.ngcsu.edu:2048/login?url=http://proquest.umi.com/pqdweb/?did=1777478451&sid=-1&Fmt=4&clientId=30327&RQT=309&VName=PQD. Accessed March 28, 2010. PQID: 1777478451.

Strychar I, Cohn JS, Renier G, et al. Effects of a diet higher in carbohydrate/lower in fat versus lower in carbohydrate/higher in monounsaturated fat on postmeal triglyceride concentrations and other cardiovascular risk factors in type 1 diabetes. *Diabetes Care.* 2009;32(9):1597-1599.

Study: moderate physical activity promotes weight loss as well as intense exercise. *FDA Consumer.* 2003;37(6):8. http://libproxy.ngcsu.edu:2048/login?url=http://proquest.umi.com/pqdweb/?did=500229001&sid=3&Fmt=3&clientId=30327&RQT=309&VNAme=PQD. Accessed March 28, 2010. PQID:500229001.

Super spices [abstract}. *Food Technology.* 2009;63(8):16. http://proquest.umi.com/pqdweb?did=1856454131&Fmt=2&clientId=30327&RQT=309&VName=PQD. Accessed November 1, 2009. PQID:1856454131.

Tanasescu M, Cho E, Manson JE, Hu FB. Dietary fat and cholesterol and the risk of cardiovascular disease among women with type 2 diabetes. *American Journal of Clinical Nutrition.* 2004;79:999-1005.

Temel RE, Rudel LL. Diet effects on atherosclerosis in mice. *Current Drug Targets.* 2007;8:1150-1160.

The truth about the China study. cholesterol-and-health.com. http://www.cholesterol-and-health.com/China-Study.html. Accessed October 18, 2011.

Tuntipopipat S, Zeder C, Siriprapa P, Charoenkiatkul S. Inhibitory effects of spices and herbs on iron availability [abstract]. *International Journal of Food Sciences and Nutrition.* 2009;60:43. http://proquest.umi.com/pqdweb?did=1828457891&Fmt=2&clientId=30327&RQT=309&VName=PQD. Accessed November 1, 2009. PQID:1828457891.

Tuschl RJ, Platte P, Laessle RG, Stichler W, Pirke K-M. Energy expenditure and everyday eating behavior in healthy young women. *American Journal of Clinical Nutrition.* 1990;52:81-86.

Tweed V. Green tea magic. *Better Nutrition.* 2009;71(7):22-23. http://libproxy.ngcsu.edu:2048/login?url=http://proquest.umi.com/pqdweb/?did=1790557031&sid=-1&Fmt=3&clientId=30327&RQT=309&VName=PQD. Accessed March 28, 2010. PQID:1790557031.

University of Georgia; study: spices may protect against consequences of high blood sugar. *NewsRx Health and Science.* Atlanta. 2008;87. http://proquest.umi.com/pqdweb?did=1542744951&Fmt=3&clientId=30327&RQT=309&VName=PQD. Accessed November 1, 2009. PQID:1542744951.

US Department of Agriculture, Agricultural Research Service. 2010. USDA National Nutrient Database for Standard Reference, Release 23. Nutrient Data Laboratory Home Page, http://www.ars.usda.gov/ba/bhnrc/ndl.

Vander Wal JS, McBurney MI, Moellering N, Marth J, Dhurandhar NV. Moderate-carbohydrate low-fat versus low-carbohydrate high-fat meal replacements for weight loss. *International Journal of Food Sciences and Nutrition.* 2007;58(4):321-329.

Vanschoonbeek K, Thomassen BJW, Senden JM, Wodzig WKWH, van Loon LJC. Cinnamon supplementation does not improve glycemic control in postmenopausal type 2 diabetes patients. *The Journal of Nutrition.* 2006;136(4):977-980.

van Vliet-Ostaptchouk JV, Hofker MH, van der Schouw YT, Wikmenga C, Onland-Moret NC. Genetic variation in the hypothalamic pathways and its role on obesity. *Obesity Reviews.* 2009;1:593-609.

Varady KA, Hellerstein MK. Alternate-day fasting and chronic disease prevention: a review of human and animal trials [abstract]. *American Journal of Clinical Nutrition.* 2007;86(1):7. http://proquest.umi.com/pqdweb?did=1302069871&Fmt=2&clientId=30327&RQT=309&VName=PQD. Accessed November 8, 2009. PQID:1302069871.

Varady KA, Hellerstein MK. Do calorie restriction or alternate-day fasting regimens modulate adipose tissue physiology in a way that reduces chronic disease risk? [abstract]. *Nutrition Reviews.* 2008;66(6):333. http://proquest.umi.com/pqdweb?did=1492541631&Fmt=2&clientId=30327&RQT=309&VName=PQD. Accessed November 8, 2009. PQID:4192541631.

Vogel JHK, Bolling SF, Costello RB, et al. Integrating complementary medicine into cardiovascular medicine: a report of the American College of Cardiology Foundation Task Force on Clinical Expert Consensus Documents. *Journal of the American College of Cardiology.* 2005;46:184-221.

Volpi N, Maccari F. Serum IgG responses to food antigens in the Italian population evaluated by highly sensitive and specific ELISA test. *Journal of Immunoassay and Immunochemistry.* 2009;30:51-69.

Wagner J, Dusick JR, McArthur DL, et al. Acute gonadotroph and somatotroph hormonal suppression after traumatic brain injury. *Journal of Neurotrauma.* 2010;27:1007-1019.

Walley AJ, Asher JE, Froguel P. The genetic contribution to non-syndromic human obesity. *Nature Reviews/ Genetics.* 2009;10:431-439.

Wang P-Y, Neretti N, Whitaker R, et al. Long-lived Indy and calorie restriction interact to extend life span [abstract]. *Proceedings of the National Academy of Sciences of the United States of America.* 2009;106(23):9262. http://proquest.umi.com/pqdweb?did=1746775661&Fmt=2&clientId=30327&RQT=309 &VName=PQD. Accessed November 8, 2009. PQID:1746775661.

Wang Y-M, Zhang B, Xue Y, et al. The mechanism of dietary cholesterol effects on lipids metabolism in rats. *Lipids in Health and Disease.* 2010;9:4.

Weil A. You (and your brain) are what you eat. *Time.* 2006;176(3):96. http://proquest.umi.com/pqdweb?did= 970371221&Fmt=3&clientId=30327&RQT=309&VName=PQD. Accessed November 1, 2009. PQID:970371221.

Weinbrenner T, Fito M, de la Torre R, et al. Olive oils high in phenolic compounds modulate oxidative/ antioxidative status in men. *The Journal of Nutrition.* 2004;134(9):2314-2321.

Weiss EP, Holloszy JO. Improvements in body composition, glucose tolerance, and insulin action induced by increasing energy expenditure or decreasing energy intake. *The Journal of Nutrition.* 2007;137(4):1087-1090.

Weiss EP, Racette SB, Villareal DT, et al. Improvements in glucose tolerance and insulin action induced by increasing energy   expenditure or decreasing energy intake: a randomized controlled trial [abstract]. *American Journal of Clinical Nutrition.* 2006;84(5):1033. http://proquest.umi.com/pqdweb?did=1191972461& Fmt=2&clientId=30327&RQT=309&VName=PQD Accessed November 8, 2009. PQID:1191972461.

West L. Which type of cookware is safest for cooking? About.com. http://environment.about.com/od/ healthenvironment/a/s…. Accessed October 8, 2011.

Westerterp-Plantenga MS, Luscombe-Marsh N, Lejeune MPGM, et al. Dietary protein, metabolism, and body-weight regulation: dose-response effects. *International Journal of Obesity.* 2006;30:S16-S23.

Westerterp-Plantenga MS, Smeets A, Nieuwenhuizen A. Sustained protein intake for bodyweight management. British Nutrition Foundation *Nutrition Bulletin.* 2007;32(suppl 1):22-31.

Westman EC, Yancy WS Jr, Vernon MC. Is a low-carb, low-fat diet optimal [abstract]? *Archives of Internal Medicine.* 2005;165(9):1071-1072. http://libproxy.northgeorgia.edu/login?url=http://proquest.umi.com/pqd web/?did=841287101&sid=9Fmt=2&clientId=30327&RQT=309&VNAme=PQD. Accessed October 24, 2010. PQID:841287101.

Wiebe JP. Progesterone metabolites in breast cancer. *Endocrine-Related Cancer.* 2008;13:717-738.

Williams EA, Perkins SN, Smith NCP, Hursting SD, Lane MA. Carbohydrate versus energy restriction: effects on weight loss, body composition and metabolism. *Annals of Nutrition & Metabolism.* 2007;51:232-243.

Wolf G. Calorie restriction increases life span: a molecular mechanism. *Nutrition Review.* 2006;64(2):89-92. http://proquest.umi.com/pqdweb?did=993103911&Fmt=4&clientId=30327&RQT=309&VName=PQD. Accessed November 8, 2009. PQID:993103911.

Wood M. Inflammation and you: how foods from plants protect us from disease. *Agricultural Research.* 2009;57(4):6-7. http://proquest.umi.com/pqdweb?did=1686383351&sid=-1&Fmt=3&clientId=30327&RQT=3 09&VName=PQD. Accessed November 1, 2009. PQID:1686383351.

www.calorieking.com

www.glycemicindex.com

Yassine HN, Marchetti CM, Krishnan RK, et al. Effects of exercise and caloric restriction on insulin resistance and cardiometabolic risk factors in older obese adults—a randomized clinical trial. *The Journals of Gerontology: Series A: Biological sciences and medical sciences.* 2009;64A(1):90-95. http://libproxy.ngcsu.edu:2048/ login?url=htttp://proquest.umi.com/pqdweb/?did=1664293721&sid=-1&Fmt=4&clientId=30327&RQT=309& VName=PQD. Accessed March 28, 2010. PQID:1664293721.

Yoon Y, Park BL, Cha MH, et al. Effects of genetic polymorphisms of UCP2 and UCP3 on very low calorie diet-induced body fat reduction in Korean female subjects. *Biochemical and Biophysical Research Communications.* 2007;359:451-456.

Zheng C, Khoo C, Furtado J, Ikewaki K, Sacks FM. Dietary monounsaturated fat activates metabolic pathways for triglyceride-rich lipoproteins that involve apolipoproteins E and C-III. *American Journal of Clinical Nutrition.* 2008;88:272-281. http://www.ajcn.org at Philadelphia College of Osteopathic Medicine. Accessed February 27, 2011.

Index

K

kale
   nutritional values, 226
   sautéing, 187
ketone bodies, 14
Koftas with Yogurt Sauce, 163

L

lamb
   Grilled Lamb Chops with Chimichurri
      Sauce, 157
   Koftas with Yogurt Sauce, 163
leeks
   Earthy Leek and Mushroom Soup, 137
   preparing, 137
   roasting, 185
leftovers, freezing, 141
lemon juice in salad dressings, 100
Lemon Vinaigrette Dressing, 99
Lemon-Rosemary Marinade, 159
lentils
   Curry Chicken and Lentil Stew, 136
   Green, with Aromatics, 201
   nutritional values, 225
leptin levels, 54
Lime Basil Vinaigrette, 107
linoleic acid. See Omega 3, 6, 9 fatty acids
local foods, vs. organic, 58
longevity, effect of caloric restriction on, 6
losing weight. See weight loss
low-carbohydrate diets. See also
      carbohydrate consumption
   100 gram limit, 12–13
   health benefits of, 12
   vs. low-fat diets, 12
low-density lipoproteins (LDL), 15, 31–32
low-fat diets
   effects of, 27
   vs. low-carbohydrate diets, 12
lunch
   eating away from home, 43–44
   nutritional guidelines for, 8

M

macronutrients. See carbohydrates; fats;
   protein
Mahi-Mahi in Raisin and Wine Sauce, 174
maintaining weight loss, 37
Manchego cheese, 215
mandolines, 112
marinades

for baked shrimp, 179
   Lemon-Rosemary Marinade, 159
   Mojo, 164
   Teriyaki Marinade, 180
Marinated Asparagus and Tuna Salad, 119
Marinated Broccoli, 116, 117
Marinated Olives and Pepperoncini, 215
Marinated Sweet Peppers and Black Olive
   Salad, 111
marjoram, 129
maternal nutrition during pregnancy, 49,
   53–54
meal planning, 14
meals, 7–10. See also breakfast; dinner; lunch
meat. See also specific types of meat
   checklist for, 64
   cooking methods, health considerations of,
      59–60
   lean, importance of, 14
   nutritional values, 141–142
   as protein source, 39
   serving size, 70
   smoked, avoiding, 59
Mediterranean Chopped Salad, 92, 105
melatonin, 54
metabolic imprinting, 53–54
Mexican Chicken and Corn Stew, 125, 138
Mexican Salsa, Quick, 114
milk. See dairy
Mojo Marinade, 164
monounsaturated fatty acids (MUFAs), 27–28
multivitamins, 68
muscle maintenance, 37
mushrooms
   Bayou Baby Bellos, 216
   nutritional values, 227
   roasted portobello, 185
   roasted white, 185
   sautéing, 188
   Skillet Chicken with Mushrooms, Onions,
      and Tarragon, 155
   Wine and Mushroom Sauce, 166

N

nitrites, 49
no-carbohydrate diets, effects of, 14–15
nutritional analysis for common ingredients,
   223–228
nutritional genomics, 54–55
nuts
   benefits of, 67